CHOLESTEROL BREAKTHROUGH

THE PRO-ACTIVE PLAN

THE ULTIMATE CHOLESTEROL-LOWERING DIET

BILL SHRAPNEL

'Bill Shrapnel has played an important role in the successful dietary prevention of cardiovascular disease in Australia during the last twenty years. This book enhances that contribution by providing a balanced and up-to-date summary of the exciting new opportunities to further reduce the risk of heart attack and stroke by improved diet and exercise habits.'

Clinical Associate Professor David Sullivan
Head of Lipid Clinic, Royal Prince Alfred Hospital, Sydney.

Author	Bill Shrapnel
Editor	Margaret Gore
Food Editor	Veronica Cuskelly
Design and Illustrations	The Book Design Company
Cover Design	Henry Bois de Chesne
Home Economist	Genevieve Low
	©Bill Shrapnel
Publisher	Ray Ramsay Custom Book Company ** P.O. Box 190, Beecroft. 2119
ISBN	1-86426-068-8

Printed in Australia by Sands Print Group Melbourne Ref. 2000

** R.A. Ramsay Pty. Limited ABN 16 001 864 446
T/A Custom Book Company

CHOLESTEROL BREAKTHROUGH!

THE PRO-ACTIVE PLAN

THE ULTIMATE CHOLESTEROL-LOWERING DIET

BILL SHRAPNEL

About the author

Bill Shrapnel is a leading Australian nutritionist whose academic credentials include a Bachelor of Applied Science, Graduate Diploma in Nutrition & Dietetics and Master of Health Planning. His career has included many ground-breaking highlights. While leading nutrition departments in public hospitals in New South Wales in the 1980s, he introduced innovative concepts of community nutrition which endure today. As National Nutrition Manager for the Heart Foundation he played a key role in the development of policy documents on diet and blood cholesterol. Bill Shrapnel is currently head of a nutrition consultancy to the food industry. In his work with Unilever Foods he has been instrumental in the removal of trans fatty acids from Australian and New Zealand margarines and, more recently, the development of plant sterol spreads - the new breakthrough in the dietary management of blood cholesterol.

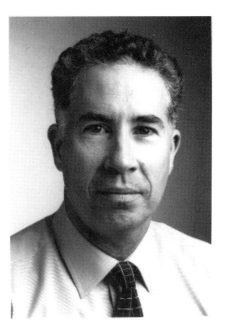

Foreword

There are many known causes of coronary heart disease, some have yet to be identified or confirmed. However, we now know that problems with high blood cholesterol make a large contribution to one's personal risk of heart disease.

In the 1980s and '90s many doctors and dietitians did not accept that efforts to lower blood cholesterol would substantially reduce future coronary risk. A series of trials through the late 1990s, conducted with gold-standard methods, have now provided convincing evidence that efforts at cholesterol reduction will safely and effectively reduce future heart disease risk. We can influence blood cholesterol levels through dietary change and/or through intake of medicines. Many people with cholesterol problems can achieve resolution by dietary means alone, especially through an increased intake of plant sterols as described in this book. But a small proportion of patients will need medicines as well, as part of a package approach.

In this timely book, Bill Shrapnel provides a comprehensive picture of the role that diet can play in reducing blood cholesterol and the risk of heart disease. He covers the full gamut of the subject from the earliest research to the latest breakthrough. Inevitably, some of the finer details remain controversial but he has indicated where that is so. For such a complex subject, he manages to present the material in a style which is both easy to understand and enjoyable to read. I commend this book to any reader looking for a practical and largely proven path to heart disease prevention.

LEON A SIMONS
    Director, Cholesterol Clinic
    St Vincent's Hospital, Sydney

Contents

Introduction   Plant sterol breakthrough   8

Part One: **The Why and Wherefore of the Pro-Active Plan**   10

Chapter 1: **Cholesterol and Heart Disease**   11

Chapter 2: **Plant Sterols: the new breakthrough**   22

Chapter 3: **The Fat Factor**   34

Chapter 4: **Cholesterol in Food**   49

Chapter 5: **Antioxidants and Cholesterol**   52

Chapter 6: **Wine, HDL-Cholesterol and the French Paradox**   62

Chapter 7: **Beyond Cholesterol: the unique benefits of fish**   67

Chapter 8: **Missing Links**   74

Chapter 9: **Battling the Bulge**   80

Chapter 10: **Variety: the spice of life**   92

Part Two: **Putting the Pro-Active Plan into action**   96

Step One: How do I increase my intake of plant sterols?   98

Step Two: How do I lower my intake of saturated fats?   99

Step Three: How do I increase my intake of plant polyunsaturated fats?   104

Step Four: How do I lower my cholesterol intake?   106

Step Five: How do I increase my intake of marine omega-3 polyunsaturated fats?   108

Step Six: How do I increase my intake of natural antioxidants?   109

Step Seven: What is a moderate intake of alcoholic beverages?   110

Step Eight: How do I increase dietary quality?   111

Step Nine: How do I eat a wide variety of foods?   112

Step Ten: What is regular physical activity?   113

Let's go shopping!   115

Meal Ideas   116

    Breakfast ideas   117
    Light meal ideas   118
    Main meal ideas   119
    Eating out   120

Recipes   121

Glossary   164
References   166
Index   170

Plant sterol breakthrough

The new millennium has ushered in a genuine breakthrough in the control of high blood cholesterol, which offers real hope to thousands of people struggling with this common problem. It's not a new chemical discovered by a drug company, but a group of natural substances found in plants, called plant sterols. The importance of this development can't be overstated. Unlocking the cholesterol-lowering potential of these natural components of everyday food will change the way diet is used to reduce blood cholesterol forever.

Scientists have spent decades searching for ways to reduce blood cholesterol in order to lower the risk of heart disease. Yet high blood cholesterol has proved a hard nut to crack. The plant sterol breakthrough has changed all this and provides new scope for people to take charge of this aspect of their health.

Plant sterols have doubled the potential of diet to reduce blood cholesterol. And, as they can be incorporated into everyday foods like margarine, including them in our daily meals is as easy as preparing a sandwich. The results of scientific studies speak for themselves. Margarines enriched with plant sterols, simply spread on a few slices of bread each day, can reduce blood LDL-cholesterol by about 10 per cent in a matter of a few weeks. Importantly, the effects of plant sterols are *additional* to those of traditional cholesterol-lowering diets. In other words, plant sterols provide a real step foward in the control of blood cholesterol through diet.

The Pro-Active Plan is the ultimate cholesterol-lowering diet – a do-it-yourself guide which combines the essential findings of the last 40 years of scientific research into diet and blood cholesterol, with the latest plant sterol breakthrough. This book will provide you with everything you need to know about plant sterols – what they are, where they come from, how they work. There is also essential information about the right fats to lower blood cholesterol, the latest on antioxidants, the role of fish in heart health and some good news about alcohol. If you have only recently discovered your cholesterol is high, this book will help you understand more about cholesterol and how it affects your heart and your health.

Many books about food and nutrition are good at telling you what foods *not* to eat. By comparison, the Pro-Active Plan is a liberating experience. Good nutrition depends on what you actually eat, not on what you don't eat. A key aspect of the Pro-Active Plan is to explore and enjoy the wonderful variety of foods available. The Pro-Active Plan is a vibrant and tasty adventure in food and an essential guide to diet and cholesterol for those who value their health and are prepared to act to protect it.

Part One

The Why and Wherefore
of the Pro-Active Plan

Chapter 1

Cholesterol and Heart Disease

When you're first told you have high cholesterol it can come as a bit of a shock. Up to this point in your life you may have been a picture of health - full of life and fun - totally in charge. Then, out of the blue, your doctor says "you have high blood cholesterol, you'll have to change your diet. You may need medication and more blood tests." Suddenly, life is a little less sure. One minute you're a person, the next you're a patient. If you're not quite ready to become a patient, take heart - there is plenty that you can do.

High blood cholesterol is no reason to panic. More than half the population has cholesterol levels above the ideal. While you should not be alarmed, high cholesterol is a serious matter and lowering it will benefit your health. The reason is simple. High cholesterol levels in the blood increase your risk of heart disease. Lowering cholesterol will reduce this risk. If you already have heart disease, lowering the level of cholesterol in your blood will reduce the chance of the condition getting worse and lower the risk of a heart attack. Is there a better reason for taking action?

The really good news is that lowering your blood cholesterol level with diet is now easier and more effective than ever before. The Pro-Active Plan will show you how. But before we consider the detail, we need to have a quick look at how the heart works, how it can become diseased and the role of cholesterol in the whole process.

The heart's essential role

It's easy to take your heart for granted. This bundle of muscle sits in the middle of the chest pumping away at about 70 beats per minute from the day you are born until the day you die. It is crucial to life. The heart's job is to supply every nook and cranny of the body with life-giving oxygen and nutrients. These are carried in the blood as it's pumped through blood vessels until it reaches every cell. There is no scope for failure. If any part of the body is deprived of oxygen, even for a few minutes, cells start to die. Performing this task is no mean feat, yet the heart usually manages it without missing a beat.

... the coronary arteries are the heart's lifelines ...

It's important to realise the heart itself is made of living cells and these need a steady supply of oxygen and nutrients too. The heart delivers these by pumping blood to itself through special blood vessels called **coronary arteries.** These are the heart's lifelines. They sit on the outside of the heart, stretched out like fingers across the surface [Figure 1.1]. Think for a minute what might happen if one of these coronary arteries were to become blocked, shutting off the vital supply of oxygen to part of the heart. The cells in this section of the heart would die.

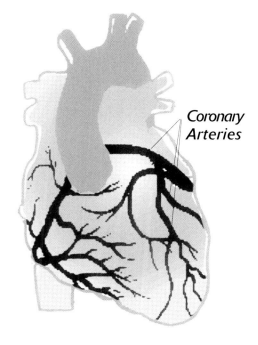

Coronary Arteries

Figure 1.1 Coronary arteries supply the heart with oxygen

What is heart disease?

Unfortunately, coronary arteries can become gradually blocked over time. This condition is called heart disease or, more precisely, coronary heart disease. Over many years, **cholesterol** and other substances can build up on the inside walls of the coronary arteries - this is known as plaque. The process is called **atherosclerosis** [Figure 1.2]. In the early stages of heart disease you feel absolutely nothing - no pain, no discomfort. As more and more plaque builds up, the blood supply through the coronary arteries to the heart can become restricted. In times of high demand, like running up some stairs, the heart simply can't supply itself with enough oxygen through the narrowed coronary arteries and pain is experienced. This pain is called **angina.**

Figure 1.2 Atherosclerosis – *the slow build-up of cholesterol on the walls of blood vessels*

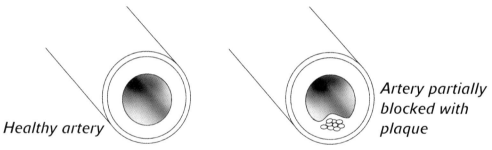

Healthy artery

Artery partially blocked with plaque

Provided the plaque on the walls of the coronary arteries just sits there everything may stay under control for years. However, this situation can change in an instant. A plaque can become unstable. Worse still, it may tear apart spilling its contents into the coronary artery. Within seconds, the situation is critical. The body's immediate response is to form a **blood clot** at the site of the damage. If this clot completely blocks the coronary artery, vital oxygen can no longer reach all parts of the heart and some of the heart's cells start to die. This is a **heart attack.**

A lot depends on what happens next. Sometimes the heart can deal with the damage and continues to beat on steadily. Life goes on. In other situations the damage is too much. The heart starts to beat in an irregular manner, then stops altogether.

What causes heart disease?

With our coronary arteries being such vital lifelines, why do they become choked with cholesterol? Solving this puzzle was one of the great medical challenges of the 20th century. As we enter a new century a clear picture is emerging.

It has long been known that **cholesterol** plays a critical role in heart disease. The presence of cholesterol in the arteries of people with heart disease was first detected in the 19th century. But how did the cholesterol get there? Was it just a natural part of growing old? Was it due to an infection? Nobody knew.

A link with diet was soon suspected. Way back in 1913 a researcher fed some rabbits a cholesterol-rich diet. The levels of cholesterol in their blood went up and the rabbits developed heart disease. These early findings suggested that high blood cholesterol was a vital piece in the puzzle of heart disease and that diet was a key.

The major risk factors

Working out exactly how important high blood cholesterol is to heart disease has taken decades of research. One landmark research study was the Framingham Heart Study (1), which commenced in 1948. It was one of the longest studies of its type ever performed. The results laid the foundations for our modern understanding of the causes of heart disease.

... here was the crucial evidence that high cholesterol increased the risk of developing heart disease ...

A total of over 5,200 men and women living in the town of Framingham in the United States took part. After a full examination involving measurements of everything that might possibly be linked to the development of heart disease, this group was then followed for no less than 40 years. Some of the subjects developed heart disease and some died during this time, all under the watchful eyes of the researchers. Piece by piece, the **risk factors** which predicted heart disease were uncovered - being overweight, having diabetes, being male, old age and more. However, three risk factors stood out from the rest as being particularly important:

▶ High blood cholesterol
▶ High blood pressure
▶ Tobacco smoking

Here was the crucial evidence that high blood cholesterol increased the risk of developing heart disease in both men and women.

High blood cholesterol

Researchers started to focus on high blood cholesterol. The picture became even clearer with the findings of another famous piece of research - the Multiple Risk Factor Intervention Trial (called Mr Fit for short) (2). The MRFIT study was amazing for its sheer size alone. In the early 1970s, more than 360,000 men were tested for cholesterol and other possible risk factors for heart disease, then followed for six years. During this time, some of the men died from heart disease. But were these deaths linked to the level of cholesterol in the blood?

Figure 1.3 *The link between high blood cholesterol and increased heart disease risk*

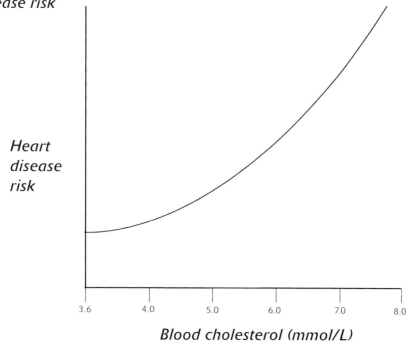

Heart disease risk

3.6 4.0 5.0 6.0 7.0 8.0

Blood cholesterol (mmol/L)

Cholesterol and Heart Disease

Figure 1.3 shows the type of relationship the researchers found. As blood cholesterol rose, so did the death rate from coronary heart disease. Importantly, there was no distinct cut-off point between high and low cholesterol. The risk of heart disease rose steadily as the level of blood cholesterol rose. This means people with average cholesterol levels are still at increased risk of heart disease compared with those at the lower end of the scale.

... as blood cholesterol rose, so did the risk of coronary heart disease ...

From Figure 1.3 we can see that the ideal level of blood cholesterol is low, about 4.0 mmol/L or below. In many Western countries the average cholesterol level is much higher, perhaps 5.5 to 5.8 mmol/L. It's not hard to imagine why heart disease exacts such a toll - the majority of people in these countries are at increased risk of heart disease.

Understanding cholesterol

Cholesterol is a natural substance and we all have cholesterol floating around in our body. In fact, the body needs cholesterol to function normally. Even if you do not eat any cholesterol in your food, your body can easily make it in your liver and does so every day of your life. Every single cell in your body needs and contains cholesterol. The body turns it into vitamin D and a variety of hormones. It's also the raw material for bile acids, which the body produces to aid in the digestion of fats.

Cholesterol is white in colour and waxy to touch. Scientists refer to it as a sterol or, more accurately, an animal sterol. It's found in all animals, including humans, and in foods we draw from animals such as meats, eggs and dairy products. As we will learn in the next chapter, there are plant sterols too. These look almost identical to cholesterol and have profound blood cholesterol-lowering properties.

The cholesterol transport system

Cholesterol is so important that nature has devised a transport system to make sure every cell in the body has just the right amount. Your liver is the "control centre" responsible for overseeing your body's cholesterol transport system [Figure 1.4]. This system is not as complicated as it looks. Let's follow cholesterol as it moves around the body.

Figure 1.4 The Cholesterol Transport System

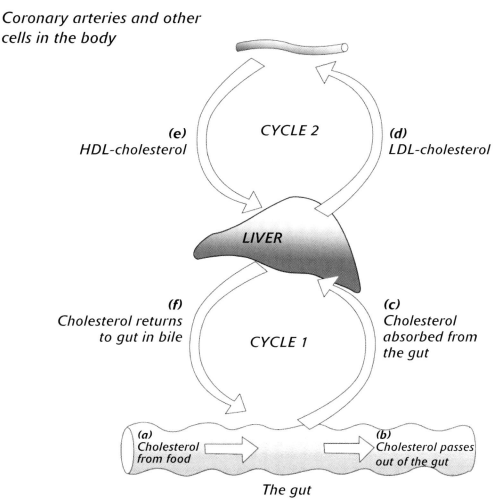

Coronary arteries and other cells in the body

(e) HDL-cholesterol

CYCLE 2

(d) LDL-cholesterol

LIVER

(f) Cholesterol returns to gut in bile

CYCLE 1

(c) Cholesterol absorbed from the gut

(a) Cholesterol from food

(b) Cholesterol passes out of the gut

The gut

Cholesterol can enter the body in the foods we eat *(a)*. Once cholesterol reaches the gut, one of two things may happen. It may simply pass straight through the gut and out the other end *(b)*. Or, cholesterol may be absorbed into the bloodstream where it is transported to the liver *(c)*.

The liver may send the cholesterol off into the bloodstream again to supply the cells of the body *(d)*. This cholesterol is called LDL-cholesterol. Cholesterol in the body's cells may be picked up and carried through the bloodstream back to the liver. This is referred to as HDL-cholesterol *(e)*. If there is a shortfall of cholesterol at any time, the liver can make some more. If there is an excess, the liver may send cholesterol straight back down to the gut, via the bile *(f)*.

Figure 1.4 shows cholesterol travels in two cycles in the body, linked through the liver. In Cycle 1, cholesterol moves from the gut to the liver and back again. In Cycle 2, cholesterol passes from the liver to the cells of the body, then back to the liver again. Under ideal circumstances, the whole system is balanced and there is no build up of cholesterol anywhere in the body.

LDL and HDL

To understand the importance of LDL and HDL you have to imagine what's happening in the cells lining your coronary arteries - the lifelines of the heart. Every now and then LDL arrives with a delivery of cholesterol from the liver and dumps it into the cells. From time to time, HDL picks up excess cholesterol and takes it away, back to the liver [Figue 1.5].

Figure 1.5 The Role of LDL and HDL – the need for balance

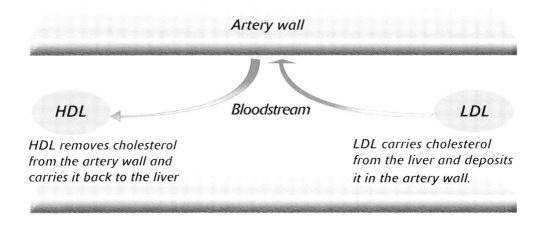

Artery wall

HDL   Bloodstream   LDL

HDL removes cholesterol from the artery wall and carries it back to the liver

LDL carries cholesterol from the liver and deposits it in the artery wall.

LDL and HDL should be in balance. If LDL is too high, too much cholesterol arrives at the wall of the artery. There is not enough HDL to carry it away and the cholesterol starts to build up. Eventually the lining of the artery becomes overloaded with cholesterol. After a while, the build-up of cholesterol starts to bulge out into the blood vessel and coronary heart disease is underway.

For obvious reasons, LDL is sometimes called bad cholesterol as it contributes to the build-up of cholesterol in the coronary arteries.

HDL is referred to as good cholesterol as it acts to carry cholesterol away from the coronary arteries and back to the liver. Whether we consider the cholesterol to be good or bad simply depends on the direction it is heading. If the cholesterol is heading into the arteries it is bad; if it is heading out of the arteries it is good.

When your blood cholesterol is high it is usually because the LDL-cholesterol is high.

Why is my cholesterol so high?

There are several things that determine your blood cholesterol level. The most important of all is your genetic make-up - your **genes**. Some people, no matter what their lifestyle, will always have above average cholesterol levels. In some cases, people have exceedingly high blood cholesterol levels simply because they were dealt a bad hand from the genetic pack. Other people may have exceedingly low blood cholesterol levels. They're the lucky ones - their risk of heart disease is typically low. If you have very high cholesterol levels, there is every chance that one or both of your parents had the same problem too.

Age also plays a role. Cholesterol levels usually rise in both men and women from the age of about 20 years and peak at about 60 years of age. Your **sex** is also important. Men have higher blood cholesterol levels than women up until middle age. Once women pass through menopause their cholesterol levels rise above those of men and stay that way through old age.

... we can't do anything about our genes, but we can do something about our diet ...

Of course, we can't do anything about our genes, our sex or our age. One thing we can do something about is our **diet** - a major factor affecting blood cholesterol levels. Knowledge of how diet affects blood cholesterol has been unfolding for decades. The first breakthrough came in the late 1950s when it was discovered that different types of fat affect blood cholesterol in different ways. Saturated fats increase blood cholesterol, while polyunsaturated fats decrease blood cholesterol. The much-hyped monounsaturated fats actually have a fairly neutral effect on blood cholesterol. These findings remain relevant today and are discussed in detail in Chapter 3.

The latest breakthrough in diet and blood cholesterol is plant sterols. These natural cholesterol-lowering substances are now used to enrich margarines and spreads. This exciting development is the reason for developing the Pro-Active Plan and will be discussed in detail in the next chapter.

Will lowering blood cholesterol really reduce my risk of heart disease?

The answer to this question is now absolutely clear: yes! For many years there were a few conservative nutritionists and doctors who were slow to accept the benefits of lowering blood cholesterol. This gave rise to the so-called "cholesterol controversy" in the 1970s and '80s. This group accepted that there was a good case for lowering blood cholesterol. However, in very scientific fashion, they argued there had never been a scientific study in which a fall in heart disease deaths had been observed following cholesterol lowering. In short, these critics demanded the very highest level of scientific evidence before they would be convinced.

... cholesterol-lowering dramatically reduces death from heart disease ...

In the late '80s and early '90s, no less than four trials were commenced in Scandinavia (3), Scotland (4), the United States (5) and Australia (6) to test whether lowering cholesterol really would prevent deaths from heart disease. These trials were hugely expensive but they provided the answer to the last big question about cholesterol. Similar results were observed in all four trials - cholesterol-lowering dramatically reduced deaths from heart disease by about 23-42 per cent. These findings led to a resurgence in interest in cholesterol among both doctors and nutritionists. The result was the return of cholesterol to the forefront of heart disease prevention. The use of cholesterol-lowering medications became widely accepted and there was a new emphasis on dietary means of lowering blood cholesterol.

The ideal diet

If your blood cholesterol is raised, the ideal diet is one that reduces the harmful LDL-cholesterol yet leaves the beneficial HDL untouched, hence the Pro-Active Plan.

Key points from Chapter 1

▶ Essential oxygen is supplied to the heart through the coronary arteries - the lifelines of the heart.

▶ A high level of cholesterol in the blood increases the risk of a blockage in the coronary arteries - shutting off the oxygen supply to the heart.

▶ The higher your cholesterol, the higher the risk.

▶ Changing your diet can reduce your blood cholesterol level and reduce your risk.

▶ The ideal diet lowers the bad LDL-cholesterol, leaving the good HDL-cholesterol levels untouched.

Chapter 2

Plant Sterols: the new breakthrough

The benefits of lowering high blood cholesterol are now widely accepted by everybody who knows anything about cholesterol. There are no "cholesterol controversies" anymore. For once, the experts all agree - lowering blood cholesterol saves lives. There are two ways to bring your blood cholesterol down - diet and drugs. While drugs may be needed by a few people, changes to diet are essential for everyone with high blood cholesterol. The good news is that lowering cholesterol with diet is now easier and more successful than ever before thanks to the new dietary breakthrough - plant sterols.

Plant sterols are a new and potent weapon in the fight against cholesterol. Scientific studies have shown they really work. Plant sterols are not a fad which will be here today but gone tomorrow. Plant sterols are here for good. Diets to lower blood cholesterol levels have been changed forever.

... plant sterols are a new and potent weapon in the fight against cholesterol ...

What are plant sterols?

Sterols are substances which occur naturally in small amounts in the foods we eat every day. Some sterols are found in animal foods and others are found in plant foods. The most common **animal sterol** in our daily diet has a familiar name - cholesterol. Every time we eat meat, eggs or dairy foods we take in a little more cholesterol. Plants do not contain cholesterol but they contain other sterols - **plant sterols**. Plant sterols are found in all whole plant foods and are therefore a regular, though minor, part of our daily diet. They have weird and wonderful names like sitosterol, campesterol and stigmasterol.

Plant sterols are "cousins" of cholesterol and look very similar to it. This close similarity in appearance between plant sterols and cholesterol is the key to the blood cholesterol-lowering effect of plant sterols.

... plant sterols look similar to cholesterol ...

Where do plant sterols come from?

Most people eating a normal mixed diet already consume about 200-400 milligrams of plant sterols every day. We eat about the same amount of cholesterol too. People who eat lots of **plant foods,** such as strict vegetarians, eat a lot more plant sterols - perhaps 600-700 milligrams per day. Plant sterols have no taste or smell and so do not affect the flavour of food. They are oily substances and occur in the greatest amounts in foods naturally rich in vegetable oils such as nuts and seeds. Cereals are not especially rich in plant sterols yet still provide up to a fifth of our intake, simply because we eat so many cereal foods. The best sources of all in our current diet are vegetable oils and foods made from vegetable oils, such as margarines, salad dressings and mayonnaise.

... plant sterols occur naturally in all whole plant foods ...

While the amounts of plant sterols we currently consume in foods have just a small impact on blood cholesterol, higher intakes can have a dramatic effect. As we will see, this can be achieved by enriching foods with plant sterols. These extra plant sterols are derived from vegetable oils, such as sunflower and canola oils.

How do plant sterols lower cholesterol?

When we eat increased amounts of plant sterols, absorption of cholesterol from the gut is reduced and our blood cholesterol levels fall. Cholesterol in the gut comes from two sources [Figure 2.1]. The majority of the cholesterol comes from the bile passing down from the liver. Bile enters the gut when we eat, as part of the digestion process.

Figure 2.1 Absorption of cholesterol from the gut

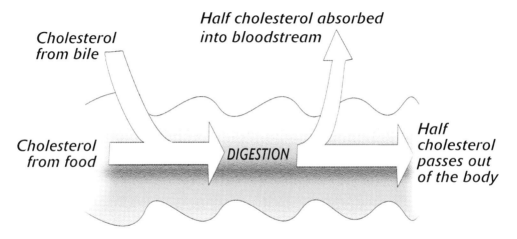

Figure 2.2 Plant sterols block cholesterol absorption

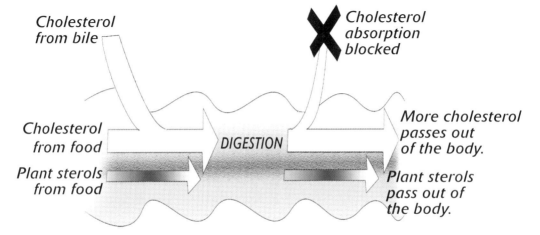

A smaller amount of the cholesterol entering the gut, about one-third, comes from the animal foods in our daily diet. This is called dietary cholesterol. Plant sterols work in the gut, where they reduce the absorption of cholesterol into the bloodstream.

During normal digestion, the body absorbs the cholesterol it needs out of the gut and into the bloodstream. On average, slightly less than half of the cholesterol in the gut is absorbed. This cholesterol then heads off to the liver. Any cholesterol not absorbed simply passes through the gut and out the other end. Wouldn't it be good if there was some natural substance that could reduce the absorption of cholesterol out of the gut? There is - plant sterols!

Plant sterols reduce the absorption of cholesterol into the bloodstream

When sufficient plant sterols are consumed, two things happen in the gut. The plant sterols outnumber cholesterol and interfere with its absorption into the bloodstream. The plant sterols themselves are hardly absorbed from the gut at all. In addition, the plant sterols and cholesterol clump together to form small crystals. Once these mixed crystals form in the gut, the cholesterol they contain can no longer be absorbed into the bloodstream and continues on through the gut and out the other end [Figure 2.2]. Overall, the body has less cholesterol to go around and the blood cholesterol level falls.

A new discovery?

With plant sterols having such a huge potential to reduce blood cholesterol, the question arises: why haven't we heard about plant sterols before? Well, nutritional scientists have heard about them before. The cholesterol-lowering effect of plant sterols in humans was first observed as far back as 1953. Scientists even observed that vegetable oils rich in plant sterols had a greater than expected cholesterol-lowering effect. It didn't take long before plant sterol preparations were available for doctors to recommend to people who needed to reduce their blood cholesterol levels.

For a while, plant sterols became a popular means of reducing blood cholesterol and they were well researched. Over 100 scientific studies on lowering cholesterol with plant sterols have been conducted. However, there were some problems. The scientists of the day had not fully unlocked the power of plant sterols to reduce cholesterol. Large amounts of plant sterols, up to 30 grams each day, were used to achieve the desired effect. Also, the form in which the plant sterols had to be taken was not very palatable. People simply did not enjoy taking plant sterols this way and interest in plant sterols slowly ebbed away.

Capturing the benefits of plant sterols

In the 1990s, researchers found that the cholesterol-lowering effect of plant sterols differed when the plant sterols were in different forms. The early plant sterols were in a "free" state. However, in nature, plant sterols are normally linked to a fat. When the cholesterol-lowering effect of this natural form of plant sterol was tested, it was found to be more powerful. Just 2-3 grams of plant sterols per day in the form linked to a fat was found to be as effective as up to 30 grams per day in the "free" form.

When plant sterols are in this natural form, bound to a fat, they can be easily dissolved in vegetable oils. This is a bonus on two counts. The plant sterols actually lower cholesterol more effectively when consumed with vegetable oil. Secondly, plant sterols in this form can be simply incorporated into any food containing vegetable oils, for example a margarine. Plant sterol-enriched margarines have now been developed and are widely available. Here was the real breakthrough. Not only had the full cholesterol-lowering power of plant sterols been unleashed, they could now be offered to people in a palatable form.

Do plant sterol margarines really work?

The moment of truth for the new plant sterol-enriched margarines came when nutritional scientists put them to the test in carefully controlled research studies. One such study was published in the respected European Journal of Clinical Nutrition in 1998 (7). Eighty people were asked to use one margarine for a few weeks, then another for a few weeks. Unknown to them, the first spread was a standard polyunsaturated margarine. The second was also a polyunsaturated spread enriched with plant sterols.

The results were dramatic - the plant sterol spreads reduced LDL-cholesterol in three weeks

The effect was dramatic [Figure 2.3]. Compared to the standard margarine, the plant sterol-enriched spread reduced the subjects' LDL-cholesterol by an average of 13 per cent. This was a truly amazing result. The simplest, easiest change to the diet, yet the effect on blood cholesterol was remarkable. Never in the history of human nutrition has a single food had the cholesterol-lowering power of a plant sterol-enriched spread. There was more good news. The subjects' HDL-cholesterol was unaffected. A perfect outcome. And how long did it take to achieve the full cholesterol-lowering effect? Just three short weeks!

Figure 2.3 Effect of plant sterol spread on blood cholesterol, compared to polyunsaturated margarine

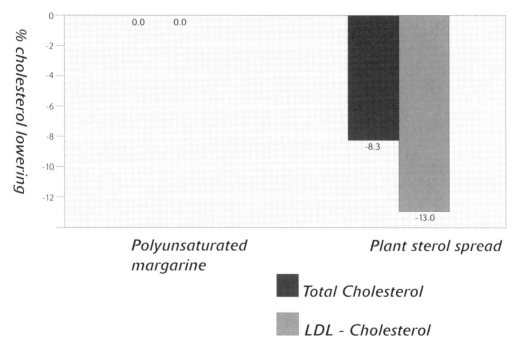

Source. Weststrate JA & Meijer. Eur J Clin Nutr 1998; 52: 334-343.

Never, in the history of human nutrition, has a single food had the cholesterol-lowering power of a plant sterol-enriched spread

A 1999 study, again published in the European Journal of Clinical Nutrition (8), confirmed the cholesterol-lowering power of plant sterol-enriched margarines [Figure 2.4]. On this occasion, the effects on blood cholesterol of margarines enriched with differing levels of plant sterols were again compared with a standard polyunsaturated margarine, as well as with butter. All the plant sterol-enriched margarines reduced LDL-cholesterol. The more plant sterol in the margarine, the lower the LDL-cholesterol level fell. However, just 2 grams of plant sterols per day was sufficient to achieve most of the cholesterol-lowering effect. This is the amount of plant sterols found in about 25 grams of plant sterol-enriched margarine - the quantity you might use on three to four slices of bread.

Figure 2.4 Effects of increasing amounts of plant sterols in spread on blood cholesterol, compared to polyunsaturated margarine and butter

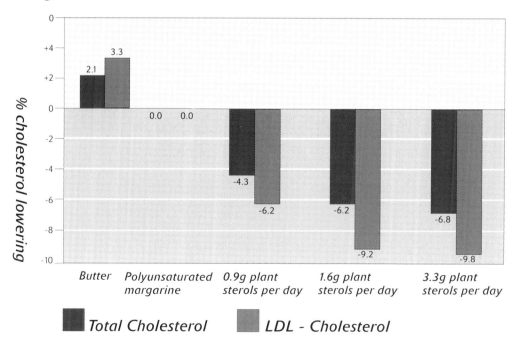

Source: Hendriks HFJ et al. Eur J Clin Nutr 1999; 53: 319-327.

Figure 2.4 also shows that butter raises blood cholesterol. This was expected because of the well-known cholesterol-raising effects of the saturated fats in butter. Changing the type of fat we eat - less saturated fat, more polyunsaturated fat - has been the cornerstone of dietary advice to reduce cholesterol for the last 30 years. However, one important finding of this study was that the benefits of plant sterols on blood cholesterol are additional to those achieved by conventional dietary advice. The implications are profound. The Pro-Active Plan is now a much more potent tool to control blood cholesterol than previous diets. Many clinical trials of plant sterol spreads and blood cholesterol are now underway.

... the benefits of plant sterols are additional to those achieved by conventional dietary advice ...

What will happen to my cholesterol?

The scientific studies showed that, on average, plant sterol-enriched spreads reduced LDL-cholesterol by about 10 per cent in three weeks. Individual people differed a little in response. Some had slightly greater reductions; others slightly less. This is due to natural day-to-day variations in blood cholesterol and to genetic differences between people. Some people normally absorb a lot of cholesterol from the gut and plant sterol-enriched spreads are slightly more effective in them. Others tend to absorb less cholesterol and plant sterol-enriched spreads are slightly less effective. Most of us are somewhere in the middle. Your exact response to a plant sterol-enriched spread will depend on these factors. When the spread is combined with other aspects of the Pro-Active Plan, a reduction in LDL-cholesterol of up to 20 per cent may be achieved.

Stop Press:
The first Australian trial on a plant sterol spread was completed at CSIRO in 1999. The result confirmed those of overseas trials. Blood LDL-cholesterol levels fell 9.6 per cent in 3 weeks.

Plant Sterols: the new breakthrough

How much plant sterol margarine do I need to eat?

In the European studies above, the subjects ate 25 or 30 grams of margarine per day which is about the typical intake for women and men respectively. Twenty-five grams of spread each day will provide an increase in plant sterol intake of at least 2 grams per day and ensure blood cholesterol falls considerably.

Ideally, your intake of plant sterols should be spread out over the day. Use the spread at two meals at least, preferably three. The plant sterols only work when they are passing through the gut, blocking the absorption of cholesterol. The more frequently you consume plant sterols, the better the effect. Different ways of working plant sterol-enriched spreads into your diet are shown in Part 2, when we put the Pro-Active Plan into action.

Are there any side effects from consuming plant sterols?

The benefits of plant sterols speak for themselves - they dramatically reduce blood cholesterol. However, we should also consider whether plant sterols have any negative effects. Fortunately, plant sterols are natural substances that are already present in our diet. Each and every one of us eats plant sterols every day of our lives without any ill effects. Those people who eat the most plant sterols, vegetarians, generally have better than average health.

Most of the plant sterols we eat do not actually enter the body. They are poorly absorbed from the gut and most of them simply pass straight through the body and out the other end, carrying excess cholesterol with them as they go. Only about 3-5 per cent of the plant sterols actually make it into the bloodstream and this is rapidly passed back into the gut via the bile. No effects on bowel motions have been reported. In fact, no adverse side effects were reported in the 100 scientific studies which were conducted in the years following the discovery of the cholesterol-lowering effects of plant sterols. Many of these studies lasted for more than seven months and used large doses of plant sterols, up to 10 times the amount likely to be consumed in plant sterol margarines today.

Prior to the introduction of plant sterol-enriched spreads, the safety of plant sterols was again extensively studied with very reassuring results (10-14). In one study, rats consuming very large amounts of plant sterols showed absolutely no evidence of adverse effects, even at doses equivalent to 100 times what we may consume through plant sterol-enriched spreads. People consuming plant sterols showed virtually no effects on every bodily measure the scientists made except, of course, blood cholesterol.

One of the things the scientists investigated closely was the effect of plant sterols on the absorption of nutrients from the gut. With plant sterols blocking the absorption of a fat-soluble substance like cholesterol, there was a chance that the absorption of some of the fat-soluble nutrients such as vitamins A, D, E and K might be reduced. Fortunately, this appears not to be the case. Levels of these vitamins in the blood were not affected when plant sterol-enriched spreads were consumed.

The absorption of some substances in foods, called carotenoids, appears to be reduced slightly. Carotenoids are natural components of fruit and vegetables. They are not nutrients and nutritionists are divided on whether they play any useful role in our health. Importantly, a study at the CSIRO in Adelaide has shown that eating plenty of fruits and vegetables counteracts the carotenoid-lowering effects of plant sterol enriched spreads (9). The role of carotenoids in heart health is discussed in some detail in Chapter 5.

The most influential food safety authority in the world today, the Food and Drug Administration in the United States, has reviewed plant sterols as food ingredients and expressed no reservations about their safety.

Suitable for people with diabetes?

Spreads enriched with plant sterols are both safe and highly recommended for people with diabetes. One of the unfortunate side effects of diabetes is an increased risk of coronary heart disease. In fact, the risk is increased by two to four times. This may be due to higher than normal blood sugar levels or by the array of conditions that often occurs with diabetes - overweight, high blood pressure, high blood triglycerides and a low level of protective HDL-cholesterol in the blood. LDL-cholesterol may be high or average. Even average cholesterol is too high if you have diabetes and blood cholesterol should be reduced. Using a plant sterol-enriched spread is a major step in bringing cholesterol down. However, the other aspects of the Pro-Active Plan are particularly important too, especially lowering saturated fat intake, weight control and physical activity. Plant sterol-enriched spreads do not affect insulin or oral medication for diabetes.

Better than drugs?

Most people with high blood cholesterol would love to be able to control it without the need for drugs. With the Pro-Active Plan more people will be able to achieve this goal than ever before. The Pro-Active Plan is the new cornerstone of cholesterol management. Many people on the borderline of drug therapy will be saved the expense and hassle of taking pills every day simply by following the Pro-Active Plan.

The Pro-Active Plan is now a much more powerful tool than conventional diets and can achieve up to a 20 per cent fall in LDL-cholesterol. Dramatic as this may be, it will not be enough for some people with very high blood cholesterol. If you have certain genes, your cholesterol level may remain too high even when on the Pro-Active Plan. Your doctor will advise you on the best course of action. If your doctor suggests you take medication, then do so. The ultimate goal is to reduce your blood cholesterol to a safe level and all means must be used to achieve the goal.

The Pro-Active Plan and modern cholesterol-lowering medication are quite compatible. The key components of the Pro-Active Plan, plant sterols and the right fats, help to lower blood cholesterol in different ways. And these differ from the mechanism of action of cholesterol-lowering drugs. Used together, medication and the Pro-Active Plan attack blood cholesterol on separate fronts and can achieve a remarkable degree of cholesterol-lowering.

What happens if I stop using plant sterol margarine?

If you stop eating a plant sterol-enriched margarine, your body will again absorb more cholesterol from the gut and your blood cholesterol level will rise to its previous level. All this will happen in about three weeks. Like all aspects of diet, plant sterols only exert their effect when you eat them.

Don't plant sterol-enriched margarines contain fat?

Yes, plant sterol-enriched margarines are made from vegetable oils and naturally contain some fat. Don't panic! Some fats are actually good for you and especially good for cholesterol-lowering. What's more, plant sterols need to be dissolved in fat to achieve their full cholesterol-lowering effect.

Key points from Chapter 2

▶ Plant sterols are natural substances already present in our diet in small amounts.
▶ Plant sterols look almost identical to cholesterol.
▶ Plant sterols reduce the absorption of cholesterol from the intestines and increase the amount of cholesterol passing out of the body.
▶ Spreads enriched with plant sterols reduce the level of LDL-cholesterol in the blood by about 10 per cent in three weeks.
▶ Plant sterols are safe.

Chapter 3

The Fat Factor

Together, plant sterols and fats are the two major dietary influences on your blood cholesterol. While including some plant sterols in your daily meals is easy to put into action, acting on fats is more difficult.

Are all fats bad?

Fat is not an inherently harmful substance; it is a nutrient. It nourishes us. Fat is a major **fuel** for the body; the other major fuel is carbohydrate. Your body is quite adaptable and can run quite nicely on a diet slightly higher in fat, slightly higher in carbohydrate, or a balance of the two. There are many examples from history of communities surviving on each of these types of diets. However, if fat intake is very low it is difficult to supply an adequate amount of fuel and people are simply underfed.

Fat is more than just fuel. Some types of fat are actually essential nutrients for the body. These are called **essential fatty acids** and they are found in abundance in polyunsaturated vegetable oils and foods that contain these oils. The fatty acids play an essential role in every single cell in the body. They are important building blocks of the membranes which surround each cell. Essential fatty acids are also the raw materials used to make a spectacular array of local hormones, which help control inflammation and blood clotting throughout the body. Our bodies cannot make essential fatty acids. Like vitamins and minerals, they are essential nutrients which must be obtained from food. We have to eat fat in order to obtain them.

Like vitamins and minerals, essential fatty acids are nutrients ... we need to eat fat

There are other vital nutrients which are both present in fat and need fat to be absorbed out of the gut. These include the **vitamins** A, D, E and K, the so-called fat-soluble vitamins. Vitamin E is an important antioxidant in the body with the vital job of protecting fat against oxidation. If you eat a very low-fat diet your intake of vitamin E and some of the other fat-soluble vitamins will also be low. Fats also help to absorb the carotenoids, a group of fat-soluble **antioxidants.**

Fats through the Ages

Fat is not a new nutrient in our diet. Rather it has been an important part of human nutrition since the days when we lived in caves. A recent review of the diets of hunter-gatherer peoples found that, on average, fat intakes were relatively high (15). However, the types of fats found in the wild foods our forebears ate were very different from those that dominate our diet today. Wild plants, fish and game animals are rich in polyunsaturated fats and low in saturated fats - the perfect recipe for low blood cholesterol and excellent heart health.

Different types of fats

Fat is not a simple substance. There are many different types of fat. The fat found in lean meat and fish is very different from that found in fatty meat. Solid butterfat not only looks different from liquid sunflower oil, it affects the body very differently too. Vegetable oils may all look fairly similar, but their make-up may vary considerably. Some vegetable oils are very rich in essential fatty acids, while others are not. Some oils are concentrated sources of vitamin E, while others have little.

Differences in the appearance and nutritional qualities of fats are mainly due to the types of fatty acids they contain. Fatty acids are the building blocks of fats. Each fat molecule is made up of three fatty acids [Figure 3.1]. There are lots of different fatty acids, though they can be broadly divided into four groups-**saturated, monounsaturated, polyunsaturated** and **trans** fatty acids.

Any particular fat molecule may contain any combination of these fatty acids. However, in fats from different sources, one type of fatty acid will tend to dominate. Animal fats, like butter, are rich in saturated fatty acids. Sunflower oil has mostly polyunsaturated fatty acids, while

Figure 3.1 Each fat molecule has three fatty acids

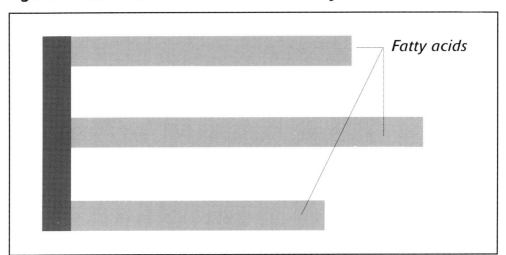

Fatty acids

those in olive oil are mostly monounsaturated. When an oil is labelled "polyunsaturated" this indicates the type of fatty acid which is most abundant, though there will still be lesser amounts of saturated and monounsaturated fatty acids present too. Figure 3.2 shows the amounts of the various fatty acids present in some of the common fats and oils in our diet.

The different types of fatty acids have different shapes. Saturated and trans fatty acids are fairly straight while mono- and polyunsaturated fatty acids are bent. These shapes dictate whether the fat will be solid or liquid at room temperature. Fats rich in saturated or trans fatty acids tend to be solid. Butter is perhaps the best example. Liquid fats, or oils, are rich in monounsaturated and polyunsaturated fatty acids. Solid or liquid, they are all fats.

Figure 3.2 Each fat has a different combination of polyunsaturated, monounsaturated and saturated fatty acids

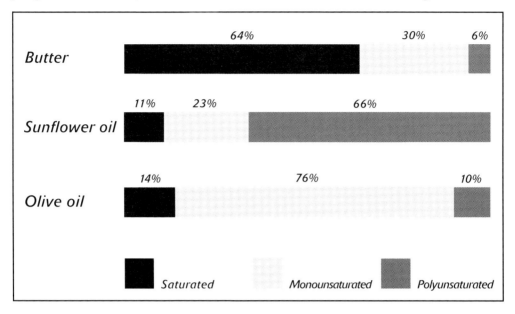

Which fats raise cholesterol?

One of the major breakthroughs in our understanding of how diet affects the risk of heart disease came in the 1950s and '60s with two series of experiments conducted independently by the researchers Ancel Keys (16) and Mark Hegsted (17). They both found that some, but not all, of the fats in our diet raise blood cholesterol. In particular, animal fats, such as meat fat and butter fat, raised blood cholesterol. Also, some vegetable fats were cholesterol-raising. These included palm oil and coconut oil. What did all these fats have in common - a high level of **saturated fats.**

... saturated fat is the most cholesterol-raising component of our diet ...

While many scientific studies have been conducted in the intervening years, none has overturned the findings of these pioneering scientists.

To this day, the most cholesterol-raising component of our diet remains saturated fat. Importantly, saturated fat raises the LDL-cholesterol in the blood.

The Fat Factor

The significance of a high intake of saturated fat on heart disease cannot be overstated. With the great many components of our diet, you would not think that one component alone would stand out as a cause of heart disease. Yet, this is the case and the component is dairy fat - one of the most cholesterol raising fats. In 1992, two French researchers, Serge Renaud and Michel de Lorgeril, published findings (18) using World Health Organisation data, which showed a clear link between intake of dairy fat and deaths from coronary heart disease [Figure 3.3].

Cutting down saturated fats in general, and dairy fat in particular, are key components of the Pro-Active Plan.

Figure 3.3 Increasing dairy fat intake is linked to higher rates of heart disease

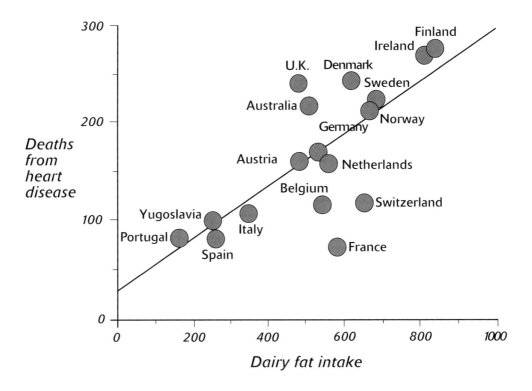

Source: Renaud S et al. Lancet 1992; 339: 1523-26.

Shows the relation between age-standardised death rate from coronary heart disease for men and women and the consumption of dairy fat (in kilojoules per day.)

More recent scientific studies have identified another cholesterol-raising villain *- **trans fatty acids.*** This minor group of fats is found in small amounts in meat fat and dairy fat as well as in vegetable fats that have been partially hydrogenated - an industrial process to make liquid oils more solid. In days gone by, small amounts of partially hydrogenated fats were used in table margarines to make them firm in texture.

Early research had found trans fatty acids to have a fairly neutral effect on blood cholesterol levels. Nobody worried much about them. However, alarm bells started to ring about trans fatty acids in the early 1990s. Trans fatty acids were found to have a double-negative affect on blood cholesterol. Not only did they raise LDL-cholesterol, trans fatty acids also lowered the beneficial HDL-cholesterol (19). These findings have now been confirmed in other studies. Around the world margarine manufacturers responded by removing trans fatty acids from their products. All the major brands of margarines in Australia and New Zealand are now virtually free of trans fatty acids.

... most margarines are now virtually free of trans fatty acids ...

Some nutritionists argue that trans fatty acids are actually worse than saturated fats, and they may be right. However, both types raise blood cholesterol and they are both bad news. An essential part of the Pro-Active Plan is to keep the intake of saturated and trans fatty acids to the bare minimum. With the low level of trans fatty acids in our diet today, the main focus is on reducing saturated fats.

Polyunsaturated fats lower cholesterol!

While Keys and Hegsted were discovering the cholesterol-raising properties of saturated fats, they confirmed another important finding: the polyunsaturated fats found in plants lower blood cholesterol. This effect, which each of the researchers observed, has now been seen in many studies. The cholesterol-lowering effect of plant polyunsaturated fats is about half as strong as the cholesterol-raising effect of saturated fats.

During the 1990s the beneficial effect of polyunsaturated fats on blood cholesterol was largely forgotten as people became increasingly paranoid about fats. As all fats were damned, people began to avoid using vegetable oils and margarines, choosing low-oil salad dressings and mayonnaise, and so on. This had the predictable effect of removing polyunsaturated fats from the diet. This shift is cholesterol-raising. If you replace polyunsaturated fats in the diet with anything, other fats, carbohydrate or protein, the effect is the same - blood cholesterol goes up.

The P/S ratio

If saturated fats push blood cholesterol levels up and polyunsaturated fats from plants pull cholesterol down, the ideal diet for heart health would appear to be one with plenty of polyunsaturated fats and few saturated fats. Among nutritionists, this has led to the idea of the P/S ratio - the ratio of polyunsaturated fats to saturated fats. A high P/S

Figure 3.4 Heart disease risk falls as P/S ratio increases

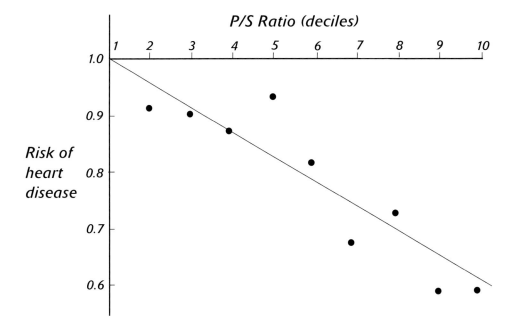

Source: Hu FB et al. Am J Clin Nutr 1999; 70: 1001-8.

Shows relative risk of coronary heart disease according to scale of polyunsaturated to saturated fat (12:0 – 18:0) ratio.

ratio (lots of polyunsaturated fats - few saturated fats) should be good; a low P/S ratio should be bad.

This concept was put to the test in one of the largest studies of its type ever conducted - the Nurses Health Study (20). The findings were published in December 1999. The P/S ratios of the diets of women were assessed against their risk of heart disease after many years. Figure 3.4 shows the results and the amazing power of the P/S ratio. As the P/S ratio goes up, the risk of heart disease steadily falls. Those with the highest P/S ratios (about 0.7) had over 40 per cent reduction in risk compared to those with the lowest P/S ratios (about 0.2).

The Nurses Health Study was conducted in the United States where the average P/S ratio is relatively low. Some countries, such as Japan and Taiwan, have much higher P/S ratios (over 1.0). Their heart disease risk is among the lowest in the world. The important things to remember in order to maintain a high P/S ratio are that intake of saturated fat should be reduced and intake of polyunsaturated fats from plants should be increased. A high P/S ratio will result.

Commonsense prevails

Fortunately, it appears that fear of fat is now a thing of the past and good science is again asserting itself over popular myth in the field of nutrition. In early 2000, the latest Dietary Guidelines for Americans were released and recommended "moderate", rather than low, intakes of total fat. A very comprehensive review of the effects of fats on heart health by the National Heart Foundation of Australia recommended an increase in the polyunsaturated fat content of the average diet (21). Commonsense is now prevailing.

Polyunsaturated fats are the essential fats in the diet, the richest in vitamin E and they reduce blood cholesterol

Polyunsaturated fats are good fats. They are essential in the diet, the richest in vitamin E, they reduce blood cholesterol and they are key elements of the Pro-Active Plan.

The Monounsaturates: magic or myth?

We can group fats in our diet according to whether they are cholesterol-raising, fairly neutral or cholesterol-lowering [Figure 3.5]. Perhaps the first thing you may notice is the middle-of-the-road performance of oils rich in monounsaturated fats, such as olive oil. Canola fairs a little better because of its low level of saturated fat. However, the polyunsaturated oils are all more cholesterol-lowering.

Figure 3.5 Effects of different fats on blood cholesterol

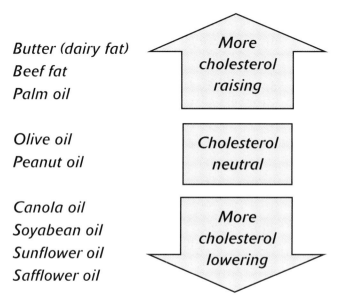

Butter (dairy fat)
Beef fat
Palm oil

More cholesterol raising

Olive oil
Peanut oil

Cholesterol neutral

Canola oil
Soyabean oil
Sunflower oil
Safflower oil

More cholesterol lowering

Monounsaturated fatty acids have little, if any, effect on blood cholesterol. They do not raise it, nor do they lower it. The neutral role of monounsaturated fats was observed as far back as the 1950s and has been confirmed many times since. This is not to say that monounsaturated fats are bad. If you replace some saturated fats in your diet with monounsaturated fats your blood cholesterol will fall. However, this has nothing to do with the monounsaturated fats. The beneficial effect on blood cholesterol is solely due to the removal of the saturated fats. Obviously, it's better to replace saturated fats with polyunsaturated fats which are cholesterol-lowering in their own right. There is a double benefit.

... monounsaturated fats have little, if any, effect on blood cholesterol ...

Enthusiasm for monounsaturated fats largely flowed from one scientific study which started in the 1960s - the Seven Countries Study (22). It showed that people on the island of Crete in the Mediterranean had low risk of heart disease. Their fat intake was quite high due to their high intake of olive oil which is rich in monounsaturated fats. Some people have claimed that the olive oil was the main reason for the good health of the people of Crete.

However, there were many desirable aspects to the Cretan diet at the time - high intake of fruits, vegetables, legumes and seafood, plus a little wine. And, most important of all, the diet was low in saturated fat. This combination was no doubt healthy but we cannot single out olive oil for all the credit. Even Ancel Keys, the chief investigator of the Seven Countries Study, is on the record as saying, "There is no proof that olive oil or the (monounsaturated fat) in it is protective other than by virtue of the fact that it takes the place of more saturated fats in the diet." (23).

More recent studies with animals have again shown that polyunsaturated oils are preferable to monounsaturated fats with respect to heart health. In what must have been a long and tedious study (24), an American researcher by the name of Lawrence Rudel fed groups of monkeys with diets enriched with either monounsaturated, polyunsaturated or saturated fats. Then he simply waited to see which ones developed the most heart disease.

Throughout the five years of the experiment, the monkeys on the monounsaturated and polyunsaturated diets had lower cholesterol levels. These two groups of monkeys were expected to have similar degrees of heart disease, but this proved not to be the case. The monkeys on the polyunsaturated fat diet had less heart disease than those eating monounsaturated and saturated fats.

The message is clear - monounsaturated fats are a better choice than saturated fats, but not as beneficial for the heart as polyunsaturated fats.

Low-Fat Folly

There was never a great deal of scientific evidence in favour of very low-fat diets as the only path to lowering cholesterol. Scientists agreed that saturated fat should be reduced, but this distinction was lost when decisions were made about how this should be communicated to the general public. Many health authorities decided to adopt a simple message - just eat less fat. After a while, all reason was lost and the public perception became "all fat is bad for you". As a result, there were some bad as well as good effects on our diet.

As some fats have a beneficial effect on blood cholesterol, it's not hard to see the folly of simply cutting fats out of your diet willy-nilly. Lowering your intake of saturated fats is fine and desirable as this will reduce your blood cholesterol. However, eating less monounsaturated fat will have little, if any, effect. Removing the beneficial polyunsaturated fats will actually raise your blood cholesterol. The greatest reductions in blood cholesterol will be achieved by replacing saturated fat with polyunsaturated fat. As a result, the optimal amount of fat in your diet for lower blood cholesterol is not low; it is moderate.

... the optimal amount of fat in your diet is not low; it is moderate ...

Very low-fat diets do lower blood cholesterol and there is evidence that they are heart healthy. However, they have some shortcomings too:

▶ Optimal reductions in LDL-cholesterol are not achieved on very low-fat diets as the cholesterol-lowering effect of polyunsaturated fats is not employed.
▶ Very low-fat diets actually reduce the level of beneficial HDL-cholesterol in the blood. Enriching a very low-fat diet with polyunsaturated fats raises HDL.
▶ Very low-fat diets increase the level of triglycerides in the blood. Raised blood triglyceride levels are another risk factor for heart disease.

None of these changes is desirable. Furthermore, a very-low fat diet is automatically rich in starch. Much of the starch common in modern diets, largely derived from cereal foods, has a strong blood sugar raising effect which persists over time, i.e. a high glycaemic index. Following adverse findings from two large research studies in the United States, some nutritionists are now concerned about further increasing the quantity of these high glycaemic index starchy foods in our diet. Radical low-fat, high starch diets may prove to have negative consequences for health, which even now we do not fully understand. A moderate amount of total fat is a safe option, the better choice for optimal cholesterol-lowering and tastes better too. Very low-fat diets are not necessary to reduce blood cholesterol and are not the only pathway to better heart health.

... very low-fat diets actually reduce the level of beneficial HDL-cholesterol in the blood ...

The total amount of fat in your daily diet does not have a major influence on your blood cholesterol level. The critical factor is the type of fat you eat. The Pro-Active Plan focuses on what is important - the type of fat. Provided this aspect of your diet is right, the total amount of fat in your diet is not particularly relevant. Lowering your saturated fat intake will ensure your total fat intake will not be excessive. Boosting your polyunsaturated fat intake will ensure it will not be too low. The result will be a moderate intake of fat.

A word about nuts

Nuts offer an excellent example of why it's important to focus on the type of fat that foods contain rather than the amount. All nuts are rich in fat and, based on this fact alone, people with high blood cholesterol used to be advised to eat nuts "in moderation" or not at all. Bad advice. Many scientific studies have shown nuts to be protective against heart disease.

In the Adventist Health Study (25), people who consumed nuts five or more times a week had a 50 per cent reduced risk of coronary heart disease compared to those who never ate nuts. Similar benefits were observed in the Iowa Women's Health Study (26) in those who consumed nuts two to four times per week compared with women who almost never ate nuts. In 1998, findings from the Nurses Health Study (27) provided further evidence of a protective role of nuts. Women who consumed nuts five or more times per week had about half the risk of coronary heart disease as women who rarely ate nuts. The protective effect of nuts was significant and strong.

... most nuts are naturally rich in mono- and polyunsaturated fats and vitamin E ...

Figure 3.6 The oils in nuts are low in saturated fat

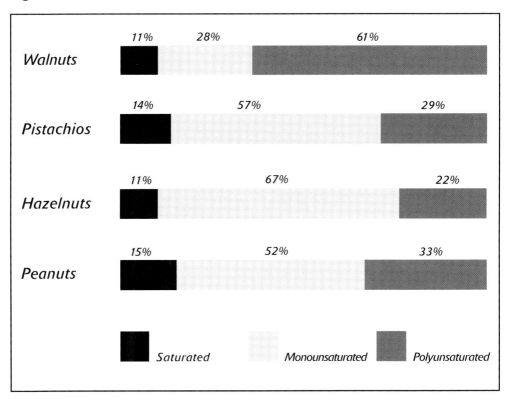

A protective role of nuts should not come as a surprise. They do contain fat, but it's good fat. Most nuts are naturally rich in mono- and polyunsaturated fats and vitamin E and low in saturated fats [Figure 3.6]. They do not raise blood cholesterol; they lower it. Logically, we would expect them to be protective against heart disease. And so it proves to be.

Won't fats make me fat?

One of the misguided ideas to emerge from the recent phobia about fats is that the only element of the daily diet that can make people put on weight is fat. If the last 20 years of research into overweight and obesity have taught us anything, it's that changes in body weight, up or down, are driven by an imbalance in energy (kilojoules). When the total amount of fuel (kilojoules) we consume through food is out of balance with the amount of kilojoules we burn off in keeping our metabolism ticking over and in physical activity, our weight changes. Certainly fat in foods is one of the body's major fuels and it's a concentrated source of fuel at that. However, in the average Australian or American diet fat only contributes about a third of our daily kilojoules. The remaining kilojoules mainly come from carbohydrate plus a little from the minor fuels, protein and alcohol. There is nothing to be gained from restricting your fat intake if you compensate by eating more kilojoules from these other sources. Fuel is fuel no matter where it comes from.

... lower fat diets coincided with a dramatic increase in body weights in both countries ...

Figure 3.7 Overweight has increased as fat intake has fallen

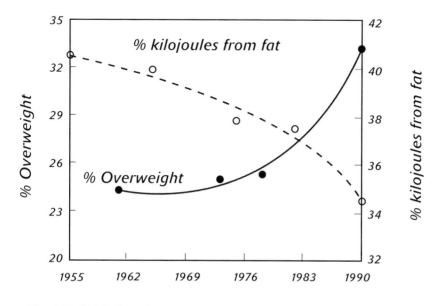

Source: Allred JB. JADA 1995; 95: 417-418.

Undaunted, some nutritionists argued that a change in the fuel mix in our diet was essential to prevent increases in body weight. A lower fat, higher carbohydrate diet was demanded. In fact, this is precisely the change that occurred in the national diets of people in Australia and the United States over the last 15 years. However, the adoption of this lower fat/higher carbohydrate diet has coincided with a dramatic increase in body weights in both countries [Figure 3.7] (28). Quite obviously, there is a lot more to controlling body weight than simply lowering fat intake.

The Pro-Active Plan is moderate in total fat for the many reasons discussed above. If you have both high cholesterol and a body weight problem, it's important that you act to get your weight down. This will help you reduce your risk of heart disease. However, we will not be blaming one nutrient, fat, for the problem. This is simply wrong and has proved counter-productive. Chapter 9 has some ideas to help reduce body weight.

Key points from Chapter 3

▶ Fats are valuable nutrients providing fuel, essential fatty acids, fat-soluble vitamins and antioxidants.

▶ There are four main types of fat - saturated, monounsaturated, polyunsaturated and trans.

▶ Saturated and trans fats increase blood cholesterol; monounsaturated fats are neutral; polyunsaturated fats reduce cholesterol.

▶ Eating less saturated fats and more polyunsaturated fats will reduce blood cholesterol.

▶ A very low-fat diet will not result in optimal cholesterol-lowering.

Chapter 4

Cholesterol in Food

So far we've looked at the two things that have the greatest effect on blood cholesterol levels - plant sterol-enriched spreads and the type of fat we eat. There are other factors to consider too. For example, cholesterol is also found in the animal foods we eat such as eggs, meat and dairy foods. This is called dietary cholesterol. But how important is this cholesterol? Does eating dietary cholesterol lead to an increase in blood cholesterol?

Unfortunately this simple question does not have a simple answer. When some people eat a lot of cholesterol, perhaps by eating eggs regularly, their blood cholesterol certainly goes up. Yet in other people there is little or no effect. How can this be so?

Are you cholesterol sensitive?

If there is little cholesterol in the diet, the liver tends to increase production of cholesterol to ensure there is enough to meet the body's needs. If there is a lot of cholesterol in the food consumed, the body absorbs a smaller percentage of cholesterol from the gut and the liver winds back its production to ensure the blood cholesterol level does not go too high. In some people this process works perfectly. In other people, the body's balancing mechanisms do not work as well and dietary cholesterol leads to an increase in blood cholesterol. This happens with about three in 10 people. These people are "sensitive" to dietary cholesterol.

... some people are sensitive to dietary cholesterol ...

As there is no simple way of knowing whether you are sensitive to cholesterol in food or not, prudent advice for many years has been to limit the intake of cholesterol from food. This advice remains sound today. This means limiting the amount of animal foods such as meat and dairy foods in your daily diet. Of course, many of these cholesterol-containing foods are also rich in saturated fats. Simply reducing your saturated fat intake automatically reduces your cholesterol intake. Eating more plant foods such as breads, cereals, nuts, legumes, fruits and vegetables will also help lower your intake of cholesterol as plant foods are virtually free of cholesterol.

What about eggs?

There are some animal foods which are not high in saturated fat but are relatively high in cholesterol or similar animal sterols. These include eggs, prawns, liver and kidneys. Do these foods need to be restricted too? On this point the nutritionists differ – some say yes; some say no. This is because any overall effect on blood cholesterol is small. Based on all the evidence, eating prawns or eggs occasionally is not a big problem. As a guide, one meal with prawns per week and two to four eggs per week are practical limits. Moderation is recommended, just in case you are one of those who is sensitive to dietary cholesterol.

Plant sterols and dietary cholesterol

The good news is that using a plant sterol enriched spread on a daily basis reduces the amount of dietary cholesterol entering the body. Remember plant sterols work by reducing the absorption of cholesterol from the gut. Daily use of a plant sterol spread has two effects:

▶ reduces the amount of cholesterol from foods which is taken up into the bloodstream
▶ increases the amount of cholesterol from foods which passes straight through the body and out the other end.

When you choose to include an egg in your meals it's a good idea to include some plant sterol spread at the same time. The inclusion of an egg in home-baked cakes, scones and muffins is fine provided they are made with plant sterol-enriched spreads (see recipes page 152).

"Cholesterol Free"

The term "cholesterol free" appears on the labels of many foods. Please ignore it. As we have seen above, the amount of cholesterol a food contains is not a major issue. Besides, any food of vegetable origin will be virtually free of cholesterol, yet it may still be very high in cholesterol-raising saturated fats. Palm oil is used in many snack foods and for deep-frying of take-aways. Being of vegetable origin, palm oil has no cholesterol, but it's dripping with saturated fat – more than lard!

If your local take-away store proudly proclaims it uses "cholesterol free" oil, make sure you ask what type of oil is used. If it's sunflower oil you can enjoy the meal. If it is palm oil you are well advised to take your arteries elsewhere.

Key points from Chapter 4

▶ The cholesterol found in food is called dietary cholesterol.
▶ The effect of dietary cholesterol on the level of cholesterol in the blood is fairly small - certainly less than the effects of plant sterols, saturated fat and polyunsaturated fat.
▶ Some people are sensitive to dietary cholesterol and show larger increases in blood cholesterol.
▶ Cholesterol-rich foods, like eggs, are okay in moderation, especially if a plant sterol-enriched spread is consumed at the same meal.

Cholesterol in Food

Chapter 5

Antioxidants and Cholesterol

The aspects of the Pro-Active Plan discussed so far are aimed at achieving one important goal - reducing the level of LDL-cholesterol in the blood. Needless to say, this is the most important aspect of the Plan. However, lowering cholesterol is not the end of the heart disease and cholesterol story.

The missing link

Nutritionists have always known there was more to discover about the way cholesterol caused heart disease. There was no doubt that reducing blood cholesterol was beneficial, but a piece of the puzzle was missing. Doctors had observed that patients with the same level of cholesterol had very different outcomes - one would develop heart disease and the other would not.

The same thing was evident on a much larger scale. Different countries with the same average blood cholesterol levels had very different rates of heart disease. For example, across many countries in Europe the average cholesterol levels were similar, yet the countries in the north consistently experienced more heart disease than those countries in the south. Other risk factors like smoking and high blood pressure did not provide the answer. Genetic differences did not explain it. There was a missing link, but what could it be?

The oxidation theory

In 1989, an American researcher by the name of Daniel Steinberg proposed a new theory of cholesterol and heart disease - the oxidation theory (29). He proposed that a crucial step in the process of heart disease had been overlooked - the oxidation of LDL-cholesterol. Steinberg knew a high level of LDL-cholesterol in the blood was a problem and increased the risk of heart disease, but he took the idea further. He proposed that the LDL-cholesterol in our blood became much more dangerous when it was oxidised, when it went "off". This added a whole new dimension to the way nutritionists looked at diet and heart disease. It meant that anything that increased the chance of LDL oxidising (pro-oxidants) would increase the risk of heart disease. Importantly, anything that protected LDL from oxidation (antioxidants) would reduce the risk.

... LDL-cholesterol becomes much more dangerous when it is oxidised ...

What is oxidation?

Oxidation is the risk we run through breathing oxygen each day of our lives. Although we all need oxygen to live, it can also cause us some problems. If oxygen gets out of control in our bodies it can lead to the production of **free radicals** called "reactive oxygen species". These are dangerous, unbalanced molecules. A free radical is a little like a hot potato. Once produced in the body it is literally too hot to handle and is tossed around burning everything it touches. A damaging chain reaction begins and continues until the free radical can be inactivated. If left unchecked, free radicals can damage everything in sight, including LDL-cholesterol. The havoc caused by free radicals may contribute to many diseases, not just heart disease.

It's not unusual for free radicals to be produced. In fact, they are formed continuously in the body every day. There are two ways to limit free radical damage. The first is to avoid pro-oxidants like smoking tobacco or exposure to UV light (sunburn), which lead to excess production of free radicals. The second is to quickly inactivate the free radicals once they are created. The body has powerful antioxidant defences in place to "quench" free radicals - to stub them out as soon as they occur and prevent them from doing any damage. Antioxidants may be destroyed in the process, sacrificing themselves for the body's sake. In some cases, wounded antioxidants may be "patched up" to fight oxidation another day.

... the body has powerful antioxidant defences in place to "quench" free radicals ...

The body has two lines of antioxidant defences. The first is a system of antioxidant enzymes, which the body produces itself. The second line of defence involves a large number of antioxidants in food we consume every day. The amount and type of antioxidants we eat varies greatly depending on the foods in our diet.

Antioxidants from fats

Antioxidants in food can be broadly divided into two groups - those found in fatty parts of food and those found in the watery part. The fat-soluble antioxidants travel around the body in conjunction with fat, get stored in fat and protect fats against oxidation. As LDL-cholesterol is fatty in nature, these antioxidants are particularly important.

... vitamin E is the most important antioxidant ...

Vitamin E is by far the most important of the fatty antioxidants and, as we will see, has a vital role in protecting LDL-cholesterol from oxidation. Vitamin E is not one substance but a group of eight related substances. The most active form in humans is the "alpha" type. Most of the vitamin E in our diet comes from unsaturated vegetable oils and foods made with vegetable oils such as margarine, salad dressings and mayonnaise. Vegetable oils vary in the amount of alpha vitamin E they contain [Figure 5.1]. Sunflower oil is one of the richest sources. Being rich in polyunsaturated fats, sunflower oil is also one of the most cholesterol-lowering oils.

Figure 5.2 shows the major sources of vitamin E in the diet. Foods naturally rich in polyunsaturated fats such as wheat germ and some nuts also contain appreciable amounts of vitamin E. Animal foods are minor sources of vitamin E.

Figure 5.1 Vitamin E content of vegetables oils
(mg alpha-toc equiv/100g)

Sunflower oil	40-60
Safflower oil	30-45
Soyabean oil	15-20
Canola oil	20-25
Peanut oil	10-20
Olive oil	10-15
Butter (dairy fat)	2-3

Figure 5.2 Food sources of vitamin E in the diet (%)

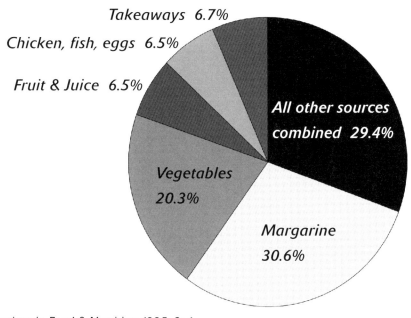

Takeaways 6.7%
Chicken, fish, eggs 6.5%
Fruit & Juice 6.5%
All other sources combined 29.4%
Vegetables 20.3%
Margarine 30.6%

Source: Perspectives in Food & Nutrition 1995: 2: 1

The **carotenoids** are the other major fat-soluble antioxidants. While not as powerful as vitamin E, the carotenoids are thought to work in conjunction with this key antioxidant. Carotenoids occur primarily in plants and are brightly coloured - red, orange and yellow. When you see these colours in fruits and vegetables you can be sure that a carotenoid is there in abundance. Lycopene, found mainly in tomatoes, is the strongest antioxidant among the carotenoids. Alpha-

and beta-carotene are found in carrots and other yellow fruits and vegetables. The other major carotenoids in our diet have heroic names such as lutein, zeaxanthin and cryptoxanthin.

Watery antioxidants

The water-soluble antioxidants are found in different foods, travel in different compartments of the body and do a different job to the antioxidants found in fats. While these two groups of antioxidants generally keep much to themselves, they also support one another. Together they form a very complicated and inter-linked defence against oxidation.

Among the water-soluble antioxidants, **vitamin C** is the best known and is found in abundance in foods like fruits and vegetables. As with other watery antioxidants, little vitamin C is stored in the body so a steady supply is required. People who smoke tobacco tend to have low levels of vitamin C in their blood, an indication of the toll that smoking takes on our antioxidant defences.

Smoking

The negative effects of smoking on the heart and blood vessels extend well beyond damaging the body's antioxidant defences. Cigarette smoke contains thousands of chemicals many of which are known to be toxic. Some of these chemicals damage the linings of blood vessels increasing the likelihood of a blood clot. Others are known to increase the risk of cancer.

One of vitamin C's important roles is to help to "patch up" vitamin E when it gets damaged in the heat of battle against oxidation. This sparing effect of vitamin C allows vitamin E to defend fats against oxidation again and again. The close cooperation between these two key antioxidants means we need to eat plenty of both, not just one or the other.

Although vitamin C has had the headlines in the past, most of the water-soluble antioxidants we consume actually come from a broad group of substances called **polyphenols**. These are found in all plant foods. Certain beverages are particularly good sources. Tea is rich in polyphenols, especially a group called flavonoids. These powerful antioxidants are about two to six times as strong as vitamin C. Red wine is also rich in polyphenol antioxidants. These substances are extracted from the skins of the grapes during their fermentation into wine.

Oxidation of LDL

In Chapter 1 we heard how the body employs LDL to transport cholesterol from the liver to the cells of the body. Throughout the voyage the ever-present forces of oxidation will be trying to rip the LDL apart. LDL must be protected against oxidation and the body knows just what to do.

Remember LDL is fatty in nature and so relies on fatty antioxidants - vitamin E and the carotenoids - to defend it against oxidation. Provided there are plenty of these protective antioxidants in the diet, there will be plenty in LDL. The body selects the alpha form of vitamin E ahead of the other forms for the important task of protecting LDL on its journey through the bloodstream. The blood itself is protective too, being rich in vitamin C and other water-soluble antioxidants.

Despite bristling with antioxidants, LDL may still be oxidised. This appears to take place at the journey's end when the LDL arrives at the body's cells to deliver its load of cholesterol. Once the LDL leaves the protection of the bloodstream and enters the walls of an artery the battle against oxidation begins in earnest.

Once LDL is exposed to the forces of oxidation the key defender, vitamin E, is the first in the firing line and the first to be lost. Then the carotenoids start to drop one by one. Lycopene goes first; others follow until beta-carotene is the last one left standing. As long as some antioxidants are present LDL remains largely intact. However, once the last of the carotenoids is sacrificed the defences are gone. The LDL rapidly oxidises. Everything goes off - first fats, then cholesterol and protein. What's left is a nasty, toxic mess.

... once **LDL** is oxidised it's not only useless, but poisonous ...

According to the theory, this oxidation of LDL in the artery wall and the body's response to it is the key event leading to heart disease. Once LDL is oxidised it's not only useless, but poisonous. Special cells within the body are called to the scene to clean up the toxic spill. They swallow up the oxidised LDL at a great rate, eventually becoming engorged with this fatty, rancid stuff . These "foam cells" are actually visible under the microscope and, when they occur in sufficient numbers, form a "fatty streak" on the artery wall and the process of heart disease is well and truly under way.

Vitamin E and heart disease

Since Daniel Steinberg outlined his oxidation theory many scientific studies have been published which indicate that antioxidants do indeed play a vital role in protecting the body against heart disease. Understandably, most of the focus of research has been on vitamin E, the antioxidant central to the body's defence of LDL.

Early evidence of a protective effect of vitamin E came from the World Health Organisation's renowned MONICA Project (30). The concentration of vitamin E in the blood of people in 12 centres across Europe, with similar average levels of blood cholesterol, was measured. This was then compared with the rates of heart disease in those districts. Figure 5.3 shows the remarkable findings of this study. In those countries where vitamin E levels are high, deaths from heart disease are low; where vitamin E levels are low, the heart disease rates are higher. In other words, vitamin E appears protective.

Another European study (31) by Bellizi and colleagues, published in 1994, investigated the links between diet and heart disease across 24 developed countries. Again, the strongest link was vitamin E. More precisely, it was the alpha form of vitamin E which appeared the most protective. This is exactly what we would expect as this is the type the liver packs into LDL to protect it from oxidation. The consumption of vegetable oil was found to be protective across Western European countries, with sunflower oil being the most potent. As we have learned, sunflower oil is one of the richest sources of the alpha form of vitamin E. Vegetables and wine, both rich sources of antioxidants, were also protective in this study.

Two large population studies in the United States have added further support for a protective role of vitamin E. Both the Nurses Health Study (32) and the Health Professionals Follow-up Study (33) found those with the highest vitamin E intakes had reduced risk of heart attack.

Figure 5.3 High levels of vitamin E linked to low rates of heart disease

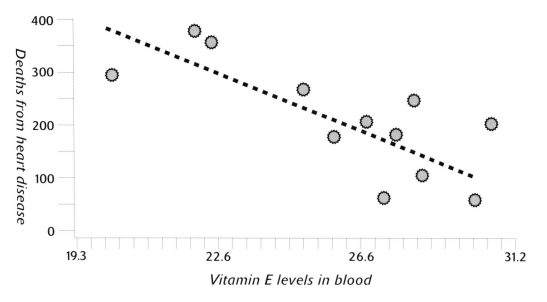

Source: Gey KF et al. Am J Clin Nutr 1993; 57 (suppl); 787S-797S.

Shows relation between age specific coronary mortality (per 100, 000) and the medians of logs of plasma alpha-tocopherol in 12 European populations.

Tea, flavonoids and heart disease

The idea that the antioxidants found in tea, flavonoids, might help to prevent heart disease is a recent one. However, some of the key evidence comes from an old and classic nutrition study - the Seven Countries Study (34). This experiment began at the end of the 1950s and continued for 25 years. Diets from 16 groups of people from seven countries were assessed and compared against their health and disease over time.

This was the ground-breaking study which established a link between saturated fat intake, high blood cholesterol and increased risk of heart disease. A recent analysis showed there were two other major factors affecting the risk of heart disease in this study. Smoking (pro-oxidant) was found to increase risk and the intake of flavonoids (antioxidants) reduced it. In the Seven Countries Study, wine was the major source of flavonoids in the Mediterranean countries and tea was the major source of flavonoids in Japan. Both areas had very low rates of heart disease.

... tea drinking was found to be protective against heart disease ...

During the 1990s more encouraging evidence appeared. In the Zutphen Elderly Study (35), high flavonoid intake and tea drinking were linked with reduced risk of heart disease. These findings have spurred new research into whether tea drinking affects cholesterol levels, prevents LDL from oxidising or protects the heart and blood vessels by other means. The results of these studies will provide new insights in the role of tea and flavonoids in heart health.

Does coffee contain flavonoids?
Coffee is not a good source of flavonoids and is not thought to protect against heart disease. In fact, the coffee bean contains two substances, kahweol and cafestol, which are blood cholesterol-raising. Drinking unfiltered coffee has been linked with raised blood cholesterol in several scientific studies. Drinking coffee also raises homocysteine levels in the blood - another risk factor for heart disease (see Chapter 8).

Should I take antioxidant supplements?

In the light of what we have learned about the importance of dietary antioxidants, a natural response may be to consider taking large amounts of these substances through pills. This could be a mistake. There is certainly some scientific evidence that antioxidant supplements can provide benefit. However, there is also good scientific evidence that some supplements can do harm.

The important thing to remember about antioxidants is that they do not work alone. The action of each antioxidant is linked to others as part of a finely balanced antioxidant system. Dumping huge amounts of one antioxidant into the system may throw this balance out. In the mid-nineties, two trials were published in which subjects at high risk of lung cancer (smokers and asbestos workers) were given supplements of beta-carotene as a preventive measure (36, 37). In both cases, the incidence of lung cancer increased. The reasons for this surprising finding are unclear. However, consuming large doses of beta-carotene reduces the absorption of other carotenoids. You end up with lots of one carotenoid and much less of the others - not the finely balanced system we're after. Early results of vitamin E supplementation trials have not lived up to expectations either.

Until we know more about the risks and benefits of supplements, the safest and best path forward is to consume your antioxidants in the way nature intended - through a wide variety of plant foods and beverages. This provides the body with a vast array of antioxidants to choose from in the kind of amounts it expects.

Key points from Chapter 5

▶   The oxidation of LDL-cholesterol may be a critical step in heart disease.
▶   Antioxidants in food help protect LDL from oxidation. The key antioxidant is vitamin E.
▶   Sunflower oil is one of the richest sources of vitamin E.
▶   Vegetables, fruit and tea are major sources of other antioxidants.

Antioxidants and Cholesterol

Chapter 6

Wine, HDL-Cholesterol and the French Paradox

Lots has been written about the French Paradox. Nutritionists and doctors have wondered for years about how the French manage to get away with it. They eat as much saturated fat as countries such as Australia and the United States and, as you would expect, their blood cholesterol levels are much the same too. They smoke cigarettes and experience the same degree of high blood pressure as other Western countries. The key risk factors for heart disease are in place, yet the French experience much lower rates of this problem than predicted.

In 1992, French researcher Professor Serge Renaud argued that his countrymen's love of red wine might explain the paradox (18). He provided scientific evidence showing wine consumption was strongly protective against heart disease and largely explained the low rates of heart disease in France. When this news went to air in the United States sales of red wine soared overnight. Rates of consumption of red wine have been steadily increasing in Australia and New Zealand too.

How could wine prevent heart disease?

Red wine is not a simple drink. It contains over 600 substances derived from the grapes from which it is made. In addition to water and alcohol, it is rich in antioxidants and also contains some vitamins, minerals and trace elements. If wine really is protective against heart disease, one or more of these substances must be doing the job. Let's consider some of the prime candidates.

Alcohol and HDL-cholesterol

Alcohol is believed to play a major protective role. No fewer than 60 scientific studies have shown alcohol to be protective against heart disease. About 10-20 grams of alcohol each day (one to two drinks) may reduce the risk of heart disease by as much as 35-40 per cent. This protection of alcohol against heart disease has been observed in men and women, in older people and in smokers and non-smokers. It is not only evident in wine drinkers but with beer and spirits drinkers as well. So strong is this effect and so often has it been observed that Professor Renaud is on the record as having said, "... alcohol taken in moderation may be one of the most efficient drugs for protection from coronary heart disease".

Alcohol is one of the few components of the diet which raises the level of HDL-cholesterol in the blood. Remember HDL carries cholesterol out of the arteries and back to the liver preventing excessive build up of cholesterol. This is a long-term effect - a slowing of the process of heart disease which operates over many years. It's thought to account for at least half of alcohol's protective effect, maybe more.

The effect on HDL is not the end of the story. When moderate drinkers cease to drink alcohol their risk of a heart attack increases quite quickly. This indicates alcohol also has rapid protective effects, different from the long-term effect on HDL. One action of alcohol is to "thin the blood" in a fashion similar to that of aspirin. It operates on the platelets in the blood reducing their tendency to clump together to form a clot. Other beneficial effects on clotting occur too. As a result the blood continues to flow steadily, even through arteries partially clogged with cholesterol. The habit in some countries of drinking wine at the main meal of the day, when the risk of a clot is at its height, may explain the superior benefits of wine over other alcoholic beverages observed in some studies. However, all alcoholic beverages appear to offer some protection.

Antioxidants in red wine

Unlike other alcoholic beverages, red wine contains high levels of antioxidants and these may explain some of the protective effects of red wine against heart disease. Like the majority of antioxidants in our diet, the antioxidants in red wine are polyphenols - similar substances to the antioxidants found in tea. They are extracted from the skins of the grapes during their fermentation into wine. These antioxidants actually protect the wine against the ravages of oxygen and help it to age.

... red wine contains high levels of antioxidants ...

When red wine is consumed, the antioxidant activity in the blood increases indicating that these polyphenols are both absorbed into the bloodstream and active in the human body. Experiments have shown that these substances in red wine inhibit the oxidation of LDL which is thought to be a critical step in the process of heart disease.

Now the bad news

With alcohol having such beneficial effects on heart disease you may be wondering why our health authorities have not been recommending a glass or two of shiraz each day as a means of fighting this modern scourge. Of course, alcohol is intoxicating. High intakes are associated with increased rates of car accidents, industrial accidents, violence in the home and violence in the streets. The cost of excessive alcohol consumption to society is well known and widely discussed.

Even inside the human body, alcohol is a good news/bad news story. While moderate intakes of alcohol have beneficial effects on our heart and blood vessels, high intakes have damaging effects on other parts of the human system. High alcohol intake can increase the risk of cirrhosis of the liver by nearly 10 times. The risk of high blood pressure is doubled and, with this, the chances of having a stroke are doubled in men and increased by nearly eight times in women. The risk of several cancers is increased - breast cancer by one-and-a-half times, liver cancer by nearly four times and cancer of the mouth, voice box and oesophagus by four to five times. Put simply, alcohol is a poison to the body, when consumed in excess.

Alcoholic drinks also contain kilojoules so excessive consumption may contribute to overweight.

The J curve

The overall effects of alcohol on health - beneficial at low intakes and damaging at high intakes - have now been observed in many scientific studies. Invariably, the result is a J-shaped curve as shown in Figure 6.1 (38). In men, as alcohol consumption increases from zero to two drinks per day, risk actually falls as the beneficial effects of alcohol on the heart and blood vessels come into play. At four drinks per day the risk is back to that of the abstainer as the benefits to the heart are offset by increased risk to other organs of the body. With further

Figure 6.1 *The J Curve - low intakes of alcohol are protective; high intakes are damaging*

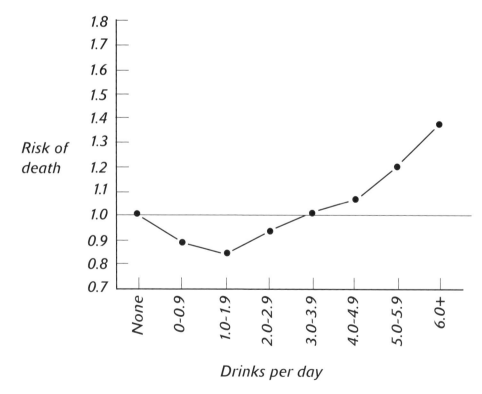

Source: Holman CDJ et al. MJA 1996; 164 : 141-145.

Shows relation of relative risk of mortality from all causes to usual alcohol intake, in men.

increases in daily alcohol intake, the risk of death steadily climbs as the negative effects of alcohol on the body start to dominate. There is a very similar curve for women with the most beneficial intake being one drink per day.

In summary, there is a "window of benefit" with alcohol. If you choose to drink alcohol, two drinks per day for a man and one drink per day for a woman is the target for optimal health. Wine may be the best choice, taken with food, in the company of family or friends. Slightly higher intakes - up to four drinks per day for men and up to two drinks per day for women are compatible with good health. Higher intakes are damaging. Obviously, drinking your weekly allocation of alcohol all in one go is not recommended, nor is drinking during pregnancy. If you have had a problem with alcohol in the past, abstinence is the best path for you.

Key points of Chapter 6

▶ In small amounts, alcohol is protective against coronary heart disease.

▶ Alcohol raises the level of beneficial HDL-cholesterol in the blood.

▶ Red wine is rich in antioxidants which may provide extra benefits.

▶ A high intake of alcohol is damaging to many parts of the body.

Chapter 7

Beyond Cholesterol: the unique benefits of fish

Although the effect of diet on cholesterol is vitally important to heart health, it is not the only thing. One food which has little effect on cholesterol has emerged with a special role in the prevention of heart disease – fish.

Interest in the protective role of fish first emerged in the 1970s. Nutritionists were struck by the low rates of heart disease among Eskimos living in Greenland, who continued to eat many of their traditional foods, especially oily fish and seal. The diet of the Eskimos was quite high in fat, yet heart disease was relatively rare.

The question was asked: was the Eskimos' penchant for seafood offering them some special protection against coronary heart disease? If so, other people eating plenty of fish should be protected too. The researchers swung into gear. They first turned their gaze to the Japanese who have traditionally consumed large quantities of fish. The Japanese rate of heart disease was one of the lowest in the world. Even within Japan, people living on the island of Okinawa, who consumed twice as much fish as those living on the mainland, had lower death rates from heart disease than other Japanese.

More positive research findings poured in. A 20-year study (39) in The Netherlands showed men who regularly ate some fish had half the risk of heart disease compared to those who ate no fish at all. In the United States, the Chicago Western Electric Study (40) also found fish to be protective.

The most conclusive proof of the benefits of fish came with a famous study conducted in the United Kingdom called DART (41). The researchers took over 2000 men who had already had heart attacks and were therefore at very high risk of having another one. One group was asked to eat more fish while the rest continued to eat little fish. After two years, the group eating fish had less heart attacks and less deaths from heart disease. In fact, the fish-eaters reduced their risk of dying from any cause by 29 per cent.

... the group eating fish had less heart attacks ...

Figure 7.1 shows the "survival curves" for the two groups in this study, indicating the rate at which members of each group died. The steeper line shows the greater rate of death experienced by the members of the non-fish group compared to the fish-eating group which was protected. Notice how soon into the study the two lines diverged - after just a few months. This indicates fish has a rapid protective effect against heart attack. Importantly, the average level of blood cholesterol in the group of the men eating fish was unchanged. It was clear that the effect of fish went beyond cholesterol.

... fish has a rapid protective effect ...

The secret: marine omega-3

All the excitement about the beneficial effects of fish against heart disease raised the obvious question: why is it so? What was the special component in fish responsible for the protection? One group of nutrients stood out from all the rest as the most likely - marine omega-3, special polyunsaturated fatty acids found in fish. Sometimes you will see these referred to as EPA and DHA. These are abbreviations of the names of individual polyunsaturated fatty acids found in fish. For simplicity, we will group them together under the one name - marine

Figure 7.1 The DART Trial - eating fish improved survival

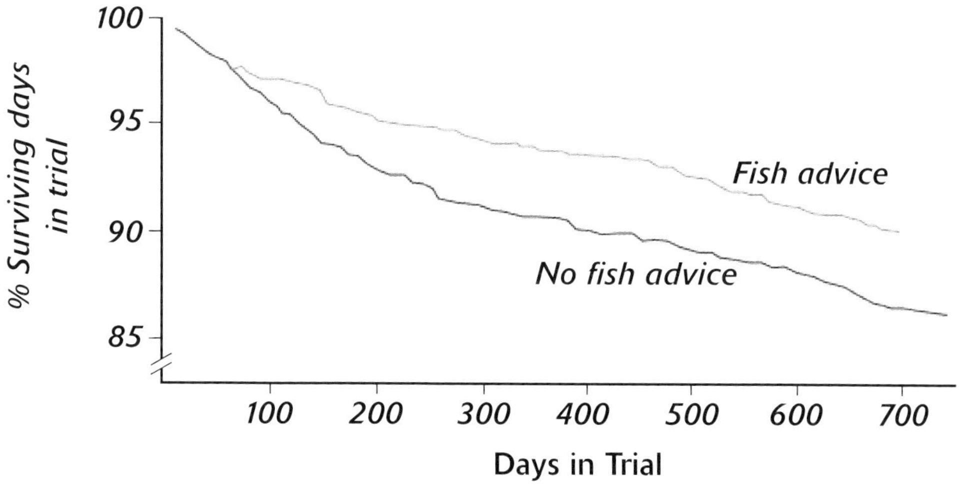

Source: Burr ML et al. Lancet 1989 (30 Sept) 757-61.

omega-3. Marine omega-3 should not be confused with plant omega-3 found in oils such as canola.

Fish is the best source of marine omega-3 and the oilier the fish, the better. As Figure 7.2 shows, white-fleshed fish such as whiting and flathead are only fair sources of omega-3; mullet and gemfish contain more; but the best sources of marine omega-3 are the oily fish - sardines and salmon. These fish are usually canned which helps preserve the delicate marine omega-3 from the ravages of light and air.

Figure 7.2 Levels of omega-3s in fish (mg/100g)

Canned fish		Fresh fish	
Sardines	2630	Gemfish	490
Salmon	1320	Red mullet	340
Tuna	260	Flathead	260
		Whiting	240
		Black Bream	220
		Ling	190

Source: Sinclair et al. Aust. J Nutr Diet 1998; 55: 116.

... the best sources of marine omega-3 are the oily fish - sardines and salmon ...

Beyond Cholesterol: the unique benefits of fish

How are marine omega-3s protective?

Marine omega-3s are not ordinary nutrients - they have wide-ranging effects. Although they don't lower blood cholesterol, marine omega-3 lowers the level of triglycerides (another fat) in the blood when consumed in sufficient amounts. A high level of blood triglycerides is a risk factor for heart disease so this is a beneficial effect. Marine omega-3 may also 'thin the blood" - a similar effect to that of aspirin, which has proven protective effects against heart disease. These unique polyunsaturated fats also make the blood vessels more flexible and more readily able to withstand the constant pulsing of the blood. Interesting as all these effects are, they do not fully explain the protective effect of fish.

The puzzle of the protective power of marine omega-3 was finally solved by some Australian researchers working at the CSIRO in Adelaide (42). They were interested in the impact of nutrition on cardiac function - the mechanical pumping of the heart. In particular, they studied the effects of different types of fats in the diet on cardiac arrhythmia (pronounced ay-rith-me-ah). An arrhythmia is a break-down in the normal, steady beating of the heart. In milder cases, this may just be the heart "missing a beat", palpitations or "heart flutter". In serious cases, the heart's rhythm can be so out of kilter that the heart may not be able to do its job as a pump. As a result, the flow of life-giving oxygen to the heart may be at risk and the heart may even stop altogether.

... marine omega-3s greatly reduce the risk of arrhythmia ...

Dutch scientists had already shown that the polyunsaturated fats in sunflower oil offered mild protection against arrhythmia. The CSIRO scientists decided to see if marine omega-3 would have any effect. The results were dramatic! Marine omega-3 greatly reduced the risk of arrhythmia. Importantly, this effect was apparent even when a relatively small amount of marine omega-3 was fed. This may well explain why the presence of just small amounts of fish in the diet has appeared to have protective effects in several scientific studies. Saturated and monounsaturated fats offered no protection against arrhythmia.

The body knows marine omega-3 is special. Unlike many fats that are simply burned off for kilojoules, marine omega-3 are treasured by the body. They sit in the membranes around the heart and from here they work their magic - steadying the heartbeat. Marine omega-3 provide their greatest benefit at our time of greatest need. When a heart attack strikes, there is a high risk of arrhythmia which may cause the heart to stop altogether - sudden cardiac death is a real possibiltiy. This is the moment marine omega-3 can stop the chaos, soothe the heartbeat and nurse the heart through its time of crisis.

Including some oily fish in a couple of meals each week will guarantee you an adequate supply of marine omega-3. This is one of the simplest and most effective dietary steps you can take to protect your heart and is an essential part of the Pro-Active Plan.

Marine omega-3 vs plant omega-3

Although plant foods do not contain marine omega-3, they do contain a type of omega-3 polyunsaturated fat. This plant omega-3 is one of the essential fatty acids and therefore an essential nutrient in the diet. Soybean and canola oils are excellent sources of plant omega-3. Nuts (especially walnuts) contain some plant omega-3 and small amounts are found in green vegetables.

Does this plant omega-3 do the same job as marine omega-3? Frankly, no. Marine omega-3 and plant omega-3 are different substances which are handled differently by the body and have very different effects.

There is much confusion about marine and plant omega-3. Much of this stems from the fact that the body can actually convert plant omega-3 into the active marine form, when it has to. However, it is a slow and inefficient process. On average, only about 10-15 per cent of the plant omega-3 ends up being converted to marine omega-3 in the body. Most of the plant omega-3 is thrown onto the metabolic fires and burned off for energy (kilojoules). This may appear a waste but it simply shows that our bodies greatly prefer to receive their marine omega-3 ready-made from fish.

The real difficulty the body has in converting plant omega-3s to marine omega-3 is seen among people who eat strict vegetarian diets. As they eat no marine omega-3, they must make all the marine omega-3 their bodies need by converting the plant version. It's a struggle and strict vegetarians always have low levels of marine omega-3 in their bodies.

Is plant omega-3 protective?

While plant omega-3 is not a great means of supplying the body's needs for marine omega-3, it may provide some protection against heart disease in other ways. In a scientific study based at Lyon (43), the gourmet capital of France, a healthy diet, including increased amounts of plant omega-3 from margarine, was fed to a group of people who had had a heart attack. The diet proved to be very protective for this at-risk group of people. Nutritionists are still arguing whether the plant omega-3 or some other aspect of the diet was the beneficial agent. However, two large studies conducted in the United States also suggest that plant omega-3 is protective. Although more research is needed to confirm benefits from plant omega-3, these polyunsaturated fats appear to be good for the heart too - not as a replacement for marine omega-3, but as a protective agent in their own right. They certainly have a place in the Pro-Active Plan.

The omega balance

Nutritionists are currently debating the importance of the "omega balance" to health. It's a rather confusing concept on which there is no consensus among the experts. Unfortunately, this has not prevented extravagant claims for health benefits from being made. There is a simple solution to those concerned about the omega balance - eat more oily fish!

Key points from Chapter 7

▶ Scientific studies have shown fish to be protective against heart disease.

▶ The beneficial ingredient of fish is a special type of polyunsaturated fat known as marine omega-3.

▶ Oily fish, such as salmon and sardines, are the best sources of marine omega-3 in our diet.

▶ Marine omega-3 do not reduce blood cholesterol. They reduce the risk of arrhythmia - an irregular beating of the heart.

▶ Omega-3 from plants are heart healthy but they cannot fulfill the beneficial role of marine omega-3.

▶ At least two fish meals per week are an integral part of the Pro-Active Plan.

Chapter 8
Missing Links

Homocysteine and folate

One of the most exciting developments in our understanding of the links between food and heart health in recent years has been the emergence of a new risk factor for heart disease - raised levels of homocysteine in the blood. Homocysteine is a normal product of the body's metabolism and is always present in the blood. However, like cholesterol, homocysteine is associated with increased risk of heart disease when it occurs at high levels. Although first suggested as a risk factor for heart disease back in 1969, conclusive evidence about homocysteine only appeared in recent years. The latest estimates suggest that 10 per cent of heart attacks may be due to high levels of homocysteine in the blood (44).

... increasing your intake of folate will reduce homocysteine levels in your blood ...

Importantly, the level of homocysteine in the blood is affected by the foods we eat. Low intakes of several vitamins - folate, B6 and B12, are all linked to raised levels of homocysteine in the blood. Put another way, increasing your intake of foods containing these vitamins will reduce the level of homocysteine in your blood, reducing heart disease risk. Of these three vitamins, folate is the most important. Scientific studies in which folate intake has been increased have observed falls in blood levels of homocysteine of 10-32 per cent.

Increasing your intake of folate is easy to do. The major natural source of folate in our diet is vegetables - yet another reason to eat your vegies! Increased amounts of folate are now present in breakfast cereals following the fortification of some of these products with folate. Perhaps surprisingly, beverages are a significant source of folate. A 1999 study by the CSIRO (45) showed that 15 per cent of our intake of folate came from drinks - tea being the major contributor, followed by fruit juice. Regular consumption of these beverages is recommended.

Stop Press: Coffee raises homocysteine

A study published in early 2000 showed that drinking coffee increases the level of homocysteine in the blood (46). Following two earlier studies which had shown links between coffee and homocysteine, researchers in The Netherlands put coffee directly to the test. In the trial, the effects of drinking either one litre of unfiltered coffee or other beverages were tested in sixty-four subjects. Drinking coffee increased levels of homocysteine in the blood by about 10 per cent. Limiting coffee intake is advised for those at high risk of heart disease.

Wholegrains: a case for whole foods?

For decades, nutritionists have recommended wholemeal bread and wholegrain cereal products as a means of supplying plenty of dietary fibre. Dietary fibre consists of various carbohydrates which are not digested and absorbed high in the intestine but travel further down the bowel where they are fermented or simply passes straight through. Wholemeal breads, wholegrain cereal products, fruit, vegetables, legumes and nuts are all good sources of dietary fibre. Perhaps the best known effect of fibre, especially wheat fibre, is its ability to promote regular bowel function.

It has long been thought that dietary fibre may be protective against coronary heart disease. However, the latest evidence suggests this story is not quite as clear-cut as first thought. The early interest in dietary fibre revolved around effects on blood cholesterol. Certainly some dietary fibres lower blood cholesterol by blocking the absorption of bile acids (made from cholesterol) from the gut. Beta-glucan, found in oats, is probably the most effective, though the effect is still quite modest. You have to eat a lot of oats in order to reduce your blood cholesterol. Pectin, found in fruits, also lowers blood cholesterol. However, other dietary fibres, such as wheat bran, have little effect on cholesterol.

Based on effects on blood cholesterol alone you would expect dietary fibre to be only mildly protective against heart disease. In fact, the protective effect appears to be quite strong. In the Physicians' Health Study (47) conducted in the United States, those with the highest intakes of fibre had a 41 per cent lower risk of heart attack, compared to those with the lowest intakes. Cereal fibre appeared more protective than fibres from fruits and vegetables. Fibre also appeared quite protective against stroke in the same study. But why was fibre so protective? Was the fibre having effects on things other than blood cholesterol?

Another explanation is that something else in the high fibre foods is also providing protection. This was strongly suggested in 1999 with new findings from the Nurses Health Study (48) which showed wholegrain cereal products were protective against coronary heart disease. The size of the protective effect could not be explained by the amount of dietary fibre present, nor could it be explained by the amount of other protective nutrients in wholegrains such as folate, vitamin B6 and vitamin E. Some other beneficial nutrient or factor may be at play. Further recent studies support these findings.

Whole Foods
The protective effects of wholegrains provide a strong argument for including more whole foods in our daily meals. A whole food is one which is consumed intact, unlike a refined food which is broken up and part of the food (and nutrients) removed. Wholemeal bread is a whole food; white bread is refined as the wheat bran and germ are removed. All fruits, vegetables, nuts and legumes are whole foods. Eating whole foods improves dietary quality (see Chapter 9).

... wholegrain cereal foods have something special to offer ...

Although the exact nutrients may not have been identified, wholegrain cereal foods appear to have something special to offer in the prevention of coronary heart disease. They certainly have an important place in the Pro-Active Plan.

Soy

Many countries consuming large amounts of soy products tend to have low rates of heart disease. This has given rise to the suggestion that soy might be protective against heart disease. The soya bean is a legume rich in dietary fibre and its oil is polyunsaturated and low in saturated fat, so soy's credentials are good. There are other components of soy which are also attracting the interests of nutritionists, especially soy protein and special compounds called isoflavones. One or both of these appear to lower blood cholesterol though the effect is not that strong. Isoflavones may also have a beneficial effect on arterial compliance - the flexibility of the blood vessels.

Although soy products are not a traditional part of the Australian or New Zealand diet, they are becoming increasingly popular. If you enjoy soya beans or foods such as tofu and soy beverages, feel free to include them in your diet. Calcium-fortified soy beverages are an excellent, unsaturated substitute for full cream milk.

Salt, diet and blood pressure

The salt controversy has been raging for decades and shows little sign of abating. There are those who argue that salt is perhaps the most important dietary factor affecting high blood pressure - one of the three major risk factors for coronary heart disease. On the other side of the fence are those who say salt is just one of several dietary factors that affect blood pressure and relatively unimportant for many people. Confused? Let's consider a few facts.

There is no doubt that salt (or more precisely sodium) in the diet affects blood pressure. If you take a group of people and reduce their salt intake, the average blood pressure of the group will fall. Based on this fact alone, it is a good idea not to eat excessive amounts of salt. However, for many people it is difficult to substantially reduce salt intake as most salt in the diet does not come from the salt shaker but is part and parcel of many everyday foods. Bread, for example, is a major source of salt in the diets of most people. Unfortunately, low-salt bread just does not taste like bread.

... the effect of salt restriction on blood pressure is small ...

Before you consider how to approach the issue of salt in your diet, two things need to be considered. The effect of salt restriction on blood pressure is small. If you were able to halve your salt intake (which is very hard to do) your systolic blood pressure may drop somewhere between 2-5mm Hg. The effect on diastolic blood pressure is less. Lots of pain, not much gain. Secondly, not all people respond in the same way to salt restriction. Some people show fairly large reductions in blood pressure while others show very little effect at all. Just as some people are "sensitive" to dietary cholesterol (Chapter 4), some people are "salt sensitive". If your blood pressure is high, you may well be salt sensitive and lowering your salt intake will provide some benefit.

... overweight is the most important factor affecting blood pressure ...

There are other aspects of diet which affect blood pressure and, for certain individuals, these will be more important than salt intake. **Overweight** is the most important of all, accounting for a large proportion of the high blood pressure in modern Western countries. If you have high blood pressure, weight reduction is a very high priority and will result in considerable reductions in your blood pressure (see next chapter). **Alcohol** also increases blood pressure, at least at higher levels of intake - three drinks per day or above. As mentioned in Chapter 6, low levels of alcohol intake are protective against heart disease but higher levels of intake cause problems. Small, regular intakes of alcohol are optimal for heart health.

Certain **minerals** in the diet also appear to be protective against high blood pressure. These include potassium, found in fruits and vegetables, and magnesium and calcium, found in dairy products. The beneficial effects of eating more fruit, vegetables and low-fat dairy products were shown in the Dietary Approaches to Stop Hypertension (DASH) study which was published in 1999 (49). The effects on blood pressure of three diets were tested - the first was a control diet; Diet 2 was enriched with fruits and vegetables; and Diet 3 contained the fruits and vegetables plus low-fat dairy products. Importantly, salt levels in all three diets were the same. Compared to the control diet, Diet 2 resulted in a fall in systolic blood pressure of nearly 3mm Hg, while Diet 3 resulted in a fall in systolic blood pressure of nearly 6mm Hg. In other words, the minerals in fruit, vegetables and low-fat dairy products all appeared to play a role in reducing blood pressure.

As you can see, dietary control of blood pressure is not related to reducing salt intake alone. It involves a combination of approaches - reducing weight, moderating alcohol consumption, moderating salt intake, choosing reduced-fat dairy products and eating plenty of fruits and vegetables. Increased physical activity will help too. All these elements are part of the Pro-Active Plan.

Key points from Chapter 8

▶ Increasing folate intake will reduce levels of homocysteine in the blood and reduce heart disease risk. This entails consuming more vegetables, wholegrain breads and cereal products, tea and fruit juice.

▶ Wholegrain cereal products contain a wealth of nutrients which protect against heart disease - dietary fibre, vitamin B6, folate, vitamin E and possibly more unidentified substances.

▶ Soy foods may offer protection against heart disease.

▶ Optimal control of blood pressure through diet does not rely on restricting salt alone. Other things are just as, or more, important. These include reducing excess body weight, moderating alcohol intake and eating plenty of fruits, vegetables and low-fat dairy products.

Missing Links

Chapter 9

Battling the Bulge

The battle of the bulge is a problem for many of us and an important issue for those watching their cholesterol. The Pro-Active Plan can help in the fight. If you're one of those people who stays lean no matter what you eat or how little exercise you do, consider yourself lucky.

All over the Western world people are getting fatter. Even in many developing countries the number of overweight people is increasing. This topic alone could fill a book so what follows is necessarily brief. In this chapter we'll consider some of the effects of overweight for the health of your heart, some of the reasons for this world-wide trend and, importantly, a few simple steps to help you regain control over your body weight.

Overweight and your heart

For most of us, increasing body weight is a concern for cosmetic reasons. It's no fun when your clothes don't fit anymore, your tummy pokes out and old friends greet you with "my, you have put on weight". While appearance is important, overweight also affects your health, especially the health of your heart. As body weight goes up, blood cholesterol goes up and the risk of coronary heart disease steadily climbs. To make things worse, the risk of high blood pressure and gallstones increases and the risk of diabetes goes through the roof.

... overweight is bad news for your health and your heart ...

Put simply, overweight is bad news for your health in general and for your heart in particular. Lowering body weight lowers the level of damaging LDL-cholesterol in the blood and can raise the protective HDL-cholesterol (50). If you're carrying extra kilos and your cholesterol is high, losing weight is an important goal.

Gluttony or sloth?

Nutritionists around the world are alarmed at the increase in the number of overweight people but are unsure about the underlying cause. The truth is out there, however. The English nutritionist Andrew Prentice put his finger on it in a forthright study published in the British Medical Journal (51). He asked whether the upward trend in body weight was due to "gluttony or sloth". Were we simply eating too much or were we too inactive?

Much to the surprise of some, "gluttony" was not the major problem. In his study, Prentice showed that the amount of kilojoules from food that people were eating had actually fallen by no less than 20 per cent in the previous 25 years. Here was a paradox - increasing weight, falling food consumption. When Prentice looked at trends in physical activity he found a very different story. Here was the underlying problem.

There's now no mystery about why people all over the world are putting on weight. In recent decades, people in modern western countries have systematically removed anything remotely approaching hard physical work from our daily lives. Lifts and escalators have replaced the stairs. We don't walk to the shops, we take the car. Rather than plough the fields, most of us now spend our working days in front of a computer. We don't even drag ourselves off the couch to change stations on the television anymore - we use "the remote". This dramatic fall in the amount of physical activity we perform in our daily lives has simply not been matched by changes in food intake. In this situation, there is only one direction that body weight can go - up!

Energy In, Energy Out

There are a thousand myths about the best way to lose weight. Before considering how to lose a few kilos, we should take a few moments to discuss how the body works, what makes weight go up and what makes it come down. Much of this is commonsense yet many still deny it in the hope that a magical solution is just around the corner.

Essentially, the body is like a machine. It needs fuel (energy or kilojoules) just to keep it ticking over - for example, to keep the heart beating and the lungs drawing air in and out. To make the body move takes more energy or kilojoules. Running, jumping or swimming takes a lot more kilojoules. Where do all these kilojoules come from? Food is the body's fuel supply. Whenever we eat food we eat a mixture of protein, fat and carbohydrate, and perhaps alcohol. All of these nutrients supply kilojoules - they are all fuel for the body. On an average day, the amount of fuel we consume in food roughly equals the demand for fuel by the body to keep it ticking over and to allow for physical activity. The energy balance is perfect and body weight is stable.

Energy In = Energy Out
(weight stable)

On some days when we overindulge, the fuel intake is over and above the body's needs. More kilojoules have come in than have been used up. The body then has spare fuel - spare kilojoules. The body only has one option as to what to do with this spare energy - it has to store it, as fat. Fat on your body is simply the body's fuel tank - a reserve of energy that the body can call on when in need. If you regularly eat excess kilojoules, the body just keeps putting them in the fuel tank and your body weight gradually climbs.

Energy In greater than Energy Out
(weight increases)

On days when your physical activity is higher or your food intake is lower, your kilojoule intake is below your needs. The body simply taps into the fuel tank and uses up a few of those stored kilojoules. Body weight falls.

Energy In less than Energy Out (weight falls)

Unfortunately, there is no simple way of draining the fuel tank once you have accumulated a big one. If you want to get your weight down, there are only two levers to pull. You can:

▶ Increase Energy Out - increase the amount of kilojoules your body burns off each day by increasing your physical activity.
▶ Lower Energy In - decrease the amount of kilojoules you consume from food.

Or you can do a little of both. But that is it. There is nothing else! There are no magic solutions; no wonder diets; no wonder drugs; no quick fixes. You have to accept this now if ever you're going to finally gain control over your body weight. The reason that so many people fail to lose weight is that they fail to accept this basic truth.

What about my genes?

Just as our genes dictate whether we will tend to have high, medium or low blood cholesterol, so our genes dictate whether our bodies need large, moderate or small amounts of kilojoules. This is not myth, it's proven fact. In a society like ours, where food is available in abundance, those people with "thrifty genes" will always be at greater risk of putting on weight. This may well explain why you struggle with a weight problem while your big-eating neighbour remains thin. If it's any consolation, your genes will help preserve you if you are ever wrecked on a desert island.

... you can't do anything about your genes, so just focus on those things you can do something about ...

Remember, you can't do anything about your genes. They're yours for life, so there's no point in cursing them. Once you accept your genes you can focus on those things you can do something about - Energy In and Energy Out. The Pro-Active Plan has three simple but essential steps to weight control.

Step 1: Upping the activity

As reduced physical activity is the underlying cause in the upward trend in overweight around the world, there will be no surprise about our first step on the way to weight reduction. You need to increase Energy Out - increase the amount of kilojoules your body burns off each day in physical activity. Just stop for a minute and think about this very important point. Unless you change your pattern of physical activity you're always going to be struggling with your waistline. Accepting the need to change is half the battle.

Once you have made the decision to increase your level of physical activity, the next issue is how? There are plenty of options and it's up to you to choose the one which most fits your needs. Activity doesn't have to be strenuous exercise at the gym. For most people, frequent mild activity is probably preferable - it can be as simple as a daily walk. If you're an office worker, perhaps you could take a short walk each lunch break and longer walks on weekends. Others may prefer to walk in the cool of the evening. Some people like to walk in the suburbs with a friend - a little moral support always helps. If all else fails, get a dog!

... every hour of television watching is an hour you could be walking ...

If you're serious about getting some weight off, physical activity must become a high priority. Like other high priority issues, it's a good idea to plan your activity - schedule it in your diary. If there's no room for physical activity, cancel something else! High on the list of things to lose is time in front of the television. Take a minute to count up the number of hours you sit in front of the TV each week. Every hour of television watching is an hour you could have been out walking. It is no coincidence that all the weight loss advertisements appear in the weekly television program.

Activity and your heart

Increasing your physical activity is not only the first step towards weight reduction, it's also essential to the health of your heart. In 1996, the US Surgeon General's report found physical activity to be protective against heart disease in both men and women. Recent evidence points to the benefits of regular, moderate activity. The National Heart Foundation of Australia recommends all people aim to be moderately active (brisk walking) for about 30 minutes or more each day on most or all days of the week. If you're not used to regular physical activity, start slowly and build it up slowly over time. High intensity exercise may confer increased benefits, though care is required before commencing such a program. Talk to your doctor first.

... start slowly, aiming for about 30 minutes of brisk walking each day ...

Step 2: Reducing Energy In

The next step on the path to weight reduction is to reduce your Energy In - decrease the amount of kilojoules you consume from food. Most people's experience with "diets" is disappointing. Everyone tends to lose weight when they start a diet, then put it all back on when they stop the diet. There are a number of reasons why this happens. Firstly, most diets usually have a gimmick to make you think that they are somehow different from all the diets which have gone before. Usually, this revolves around identifying one particular nutrient in the diet as the villain, then removing it from the diet. Back in the 1970s, carbohydrate was the villain - fat was fine.

During the 1980s and '90s, the weight control diet in vogue was the exact opposite - low in fat, but high in carbohydrate. Fat was the villain this time. Such was the faith in the low-fat approach to weight reduction that the populations of Australia and the United States were advised to follow this path in recent years. Significant falls in the fat content of the national diets have resulted. Unfortunately, the average body weights in both countries have shot up dramatically during the same period (28). Health authorities in the United States are now referring to the "unintended consequences" of the "eat less fat" message. Those consequences are that Americans have eaten more sugar, eaten more kilojoules and become fatter!

The truth is that there have been no breakthroughs in weight control in recent decades and they are unlikely to ever happen. Gimmicky high-this, low-that diets are not the key to losing weight. Weight control through food requires one simple thing - reduce Energy In. This can be achieved in a number of ways. It's best to find one that suits you as an individual.

The time factor

Another reason for the disappointment with diets has to do with time. The focus of many diets is often a week or two. Any effect on weight during this time may appear to be impressive, but time and time again people see their weight return to previous levels. The reason is simple: the meals you eat week after week, month after month are the ones that count. This is what determines your real Energy In. Foods you eat (or don't eat) over a two-week period of diet have little impact on your weight in the long-term.

The focus of weight control on the Pro-Active Plan is long-term. It's all about what you eat every day of your life, not what you eat in a few painful weeks here and there. We don't aim for a dramatic decrease in weight in a few days; we aim for sustainable weight loss. Our approach will not include a huge reduction in the kilojoules you eat - nobody can maintain this for very long. Rather, the aim is to reduce your current kilojoule intake by about 10-15 per cent. This, combined with increased activity levels, will be sufficient to commence and sustain weight loss.

... the aim is to reduce your current kilojoule intake by about 10-15 per cent ...

Reducing your current kilojoule intake by 10-15 per cent isn't hard and there's no need to count kilojoules, count fats, count anything. Our approach is a simple one - improve dietary quality; establish the right meal pattern; then stick with it, for good. The focus is long-term. Slow and steady wins the race.

Improving dietary quality

The choice of food and drink to include in your daily meals is governed by the need to achieve two goals:

▶ Reduce Energy In
▶ Maintain or increase intake of essential nutrients

At first glance this may appear hard to do. When we eat food we consume kilojoules and nutrients. When we eat more food we take in more kilojoules and more nutrients. But how can we eat less kilojoules and more nutrients?

The answer lies in changing the mix of foods we eat - eating less of the troublesome foods to save some kilojoules and replacing these with more highly nutritious foods to boost nutrient intake. In other words we need to improve dietary quality.

There are four key changes to make to improve dietary quality:

▶ Reduce saturated fat intake.

Choosing foods low in saturated fat to reduce blood cholesterol will remove useless kilojoules from your daily diet - lean meat has less kilojoules than fatty meat; skim milk has less kilojoules than full cream; steering clear of those pastries, biscuits and snack foods will also help. Bypassing take-aways, dripping with saturated fat, will bypass plenty of kilojoules too.

▶ Reduce intake of "empty" kilojoules.

"Empty" kilojoules are those which come with no other nutrients at all. The advice here can be reduced to three words - skip the sugar! While sugar has no effect on blood cholesterol, it's the most useless of all the components of your daily diet if you're watching your weight. It's not "pure, white and deadly" as some have claimed, just useless. When your overall kilojoule intake is reduced, you need to make sure your body is getting full value from those kilojoules it gets, i.e. plenty of nutrients. Pure sugar provides unwanted kilojoules but no worthwhile nutrients whatsoever. Everything else you eat will have at least a handful of nutrients to offer your body. But not sugar. Every atom of goodness has been refined out of it.

But be realistic. A little sugar here and there, perhaps to provide some flavour to wholegrain breakfast cereals, is not a problem. Unfortunately, sugar is often consumed all by itself in large quantities, especially in soft drinks. A 1999 report by the CSIRO (45) showed that 15 per cent of the kilojoules we consume don't come from foods at all, but from beverages. In fact, 36 per cent of our total sugar intake came from soft drinks.

As a general rule, kilojoules should be eaten, not drunk. This goes for alcoholic drinks as well. One or two drinks will give you the protective effect discussed in Chapter 6. Any further drinks are just more fuel for the fuel tank - unwanted kilojoules leading to unwanted kilos.

Does alcohol help you slim?

Although alcohol contains kilojoules, for years some nutritionists have argued that kilojoules from alcohol don't contribute their fair share to body weight. This was based on observed links between slimness and alcohol intake. The implication was - drink alcohol, stay slim. While an attractive theory for some, sophisticated studies have now proven it not to be true. Alcohol kilojoules count!

▶ Choose more whole foods.

There are many occasions where similar foods, with similar kilojoules, are on offer, yet one is richer in nutrients than the offer. Cereal products are perhaps the best example. A slice of wholemeal bread contains nutrients and fibre from the germ and the bran of the wheat grain plus the starchy centre. A slice of white bread contains nutrients from the starchy part. The whole food has more to offer.

The choices among breakfast cereals are even more stark. In this case, some highly refined starchy cereals may contain up to 40 per cent sugar. How does this compare with wholewheat cereals with all their nutrients and fibre? As we saw in the last chapter, wholegrain cereal products may have a special protective role against heart disease.

Other whole foods include nuts, legumes, vegetables and fruits. As we will see below, vegetables have another special role to play for those watching their weight.

▶   Choose more low kilojoule, high bulk foods.

If only there was a group of foods which did not contain too many kilojoules, was high in bulk to fill you up and was rich in nutrients as well. There is - vegetables. With the exception of potatoes, here's a group of foods you can eat in quantity. Increasing vegetable intake is a key element of weight control and an essential part of all midday and evening meals.

Step 3: How to eat

The Pro-Active Plan offers plenty of options on what to eat. However, half the battle of losing weight is all about how to eat - achieving a pattern of eating (and drinking) which will lead to long-term weight loss without the discomfort of excessive hunger. It involves changing the way we eat, perhaps changing the times we eat and managing the signals that trigger us to eat. There is no pattern which suits all people. Here are a few simple steps which you may find helpful to achieve a weight-reducing pattern:

▶   **Eat three meals a day, including breakfast**
▶   **Eat nothing between meals**
▶   **Eat a small evening meal, with plenty of vegetables**
▶   **Don't eat standing up**

The three meals system ensures you get adequate opportunity to enjoy the foods your body needs. It's important to nourish your body well during weight reduction, not deprive it of the very nutrients it needs to function. Don't try to starve yourself. Avoiding between-meal snacks will help to clear away those kilojoules we need to lose. Your meals will also be sufficiently spaced to allow your hunger to come into play before each meal. And you should feel hungry at meal time. Traditionally, the evening meal is the largest meal of the day for most people. It's also taken when your body's need for kilojoules is about to fall as you head off to bed. Having a smaller dinner will help you trim off some of those kilojoules and ensure you'll be feeling peckish at breakfast time. If you're not hungry first thing in the morning it's usually because of the large meal you had the night before.

Importantly, sit down when you eat. This is not simply so that you can take a little time to relax and savour your food, though this is important. The idea is to ensure you limit your eating to meal times. Many overweight people arrive at the dinner table and say "I'm just not hungry". The reason is that they have been inadvertently eating all afternoon - grabbing a snack on the run down to the shops, a few biscuits to keep going, nibbling during meal preparation and so on. Train yourself to ask the question every time you put food to your mouth: Am I standing up? If so, this is not the time to eat. If you have to eat, then sit down, make a meal of it and enjoy it.

The Joy of Food

Food is one of the great joys of life. We celebrate at the table; we romance at the table; we socialise at the table. Is it possible to continue to enjoy these aspects of food and lose weight too? Of course it is. One of the problems with "diets" is that people inevitably break them, by going out and having fun. They then feel depressed at their failure and give weight control away. Rather than setting yourself up for failure, assume there will be some meals which fall short of ideal. Rather than punishing youself, just re-focus on your goals and set things right at the next meal. One meal has little influence on your body weight. The total of all the other meals will determine which way your weight is heading.

Training your stomach

Reducing your Energy In and increasing your Energy Out is not going to happen without a fuss. Your body will have less kilojoules coming in than it needs and will have to call on your energy reserves - the fat on your body. However, the change will not go unnoticed. In fact, one part of your anatomy is going to complain - your stomach. Your stomach is used to how much food it expects to receive and when to expect it. If you change anything your stomach will tell you all about it. Initially, you will feel hungry. Real hunger is one of those things that many of us seldom experience, yet pangs of hunger are actually a good sign. The body is saying "I'm out of fuel. I'm calling on my reserves". Hunger is the feeling of losing weight.

... *hunger is the feeling of losing weight* ...

Hunger is also a very uncomfortable feeling which needs to be managed carefully. You know when you're on the right track when you feel hungry at meal time, satisfied afterwards, then hungry again by the next meal. This is the natural rhythm which many of us have lost. To win it back requires a little training. Your stomach will take some time to get used to your new meal pattern and the amounts of food you eat. This does not take long - usually about a week.

Key points from Chapter 9

▶ Being overweight is bad for your heart.

▶ There's no simple solution to overweight. It takes time and persistence to permanently lose weight.

▶ A low level of physical activity is a major underlying cause of overweight. Getting moderate, regular physical activity is the first step to long-term weight control.

▶ Short-term diets are not a solution to weight control. A long-term approach to food is essential.

▶ Improve dietary quality by reducing intake of saturated fat and sugar, choose more wholegrain cereals and eat plenty of vegetables.

▶ Establish a meal pattern which balances good nutrition with hunger and feeling satisfied.

Chapter 10

Variety: the spice of life

Many books about food and nutrition are good at telling you what foods not to eat. By comparison, the Pro-Active Plan is a liberating experience. Certainly, we have to limit the intake of some foods. After all, we need to reduce the intake of those foods that are dripping with cholesterol-raising saturated fats. However, we also need to ensure that the daily diet does more than just lower your cholesterol. It needs to be a vibrant diet that optimises heart health through food. Simply cutting out foods from your daily diet runs counter to one of the fundamental principles of good nutrition - to eat a wide variety of foods. Good nutrition depends on what you actually eat, not on what you don't eat. One important aspect of the Pro-Active Plan is to broaden the range of foods in your meals, not restrict it.

... good nutrition depends on what you actually eat, not on what you don't eat ...

The importance of variety

Variety is vital to good nutrition. Each food has a unique array of nutrients and often something special to offer. The best sources of calcium in our diet are dairy products. Fruits have plenty of vitamin C. Vegetable oils provide most of our vitamin E. Meat has plenty of iron and zinc. Vegetables contain folate. Cereal products are rich in

B vitamins and fibre. Fish contains those special polyunsaturated fats. The antioxidant lycopene is primarily found in tomatoes and so it goes on. Every food has something to contribute to health and wellbeing, yet no food has everything you need. There are no wonder foods. Rather, different foods all have a small part to play. Together, they deliver the full symphony. Obviously, the wider the variety of foods in your daily meals, the more likely you are to benefit from the bounty on offer. If your food selection is narrow, there is increased chance that you'll have too little of some important nutrients and perhaps too much of some things which you do not need - like saturated fat.

Benefits of plant foods

Plant foods are natural sources of plant sterols but contain virtually no cholesterol. With just a few exceptions, plant foods are also low in saturated fat. The potential variety is enormous, yet most people usually confine themselves to a fairly narrow range of plant foods. Think about your own diet for a minute. Do you eat bread and other cereal foods each day? The answer is probably yes because these are very common in our diet. But how many vegetables do you eat each day? What about fruit? Are you one of the four in 10 adults who don't eat a single piece of fruit each day? How many times a week do you eat nuts? What about legumes? How many of these different classes of plant foods find their way into you diet each day, or each week?

... four in 10 adults do not eat a single piece of fruit each day ...

The variety of plant foods available is vast, so take advantage of it. The recipes in Part 2 of the Pro-Active Plan may give you some fresh ideas on how to include a few new plant foods in your daily meals.

Are animal foods okay?

Foods of animal origin, especially meat and dairy products, are rich in saturated fats and therefore foods to watch. Sometimes animal foods are portrayed as "bad" for you and recommended for deletion from the daily diet. This is not the way to go. Only the fat in these foods causes a problem - the remainder of these foods is loaded with nutrients and very nutritious.

The Pro-Active Plan includes a variety of both animal and plant foods. Some people may choose not to include foods of animal origin in their diet for a variety of personal reasons. However, from a purely nutritional point of view, restricting yourself to just one half of the food kingdom is neither necessary nor desirable. Animal foods have plenty to offer and can cover some of the shortcomings of vegetable foods. For example, the type of iron found in meat is more easily absorbed from the gut than the type of iron found in foods of vegetable origin. No plant food contributes as much calcium in the diet as milk. The special polyunsaturated fats found in fish are simply not found in our plant foods. Strict vegetarians make do by making some of these fats in their bodies. However, the levels of these polyunsaturates in the blood of vegetarians never reach the levels of those who regularly consume fish.

Choosing animal foods on the Pro-Active Plan is straightforward - choose low-fat versions. Take the fat out of dairy products and you take out the problem. Low-fat milk and yoghurt are fine and should find a place in your daily diet. Lean meat has little saturated fat but virtually all of the valuable nutrients for which meat is renowned. Chicken can be quite fatty, but some lean chicken breast stir-fried in a little healthy sunflower oil does not present a problem. Most fish are naturally low in fat and the fat they contain is good polyunsaturated fat. All these "animal" foods can find a place in the Pro-Active Plan.

Tasty cuisines

A key aspect of the Pro-Active Plan is to explore and enjoy the wonderful variety of foods available. As a first step, try dishes from different national cuisines which incorporate foods that may not be a standard part of your daily meals. Two inspiring cuisines are modern Asian and traditional Mediterranean. Although there are many differences between these two cuisines, they share important things in common - a low content of saturated fat, use of unsaturated vegetable oils, plenty of cereals, plenty of fish and lots of vegetables - all key elements of the Pro-Active Plan. Most importantly, they taste great and provide endless delights at the dinner table at home or out at a restaurant. Rest assured, the Pro-Active Plan is not a boring "diet"; it's an adventure.

Key points from Chapter 10

▶ Eating a wide variety of foods is a fundamental principle of good nutrition.

▶ All foods have useful nutrients to offer.

▶ Plant foods are highly recommended.

▶ For optimal nutrition, a combination of plant and animal foods is required.

Part Two

Putting the Pro-Active
Plan into Action

In Part 1 of this book we journeyed through the latest scientific information on the effects of diet on blood cholesterol and other aspects of heart health. For our new knowledge to do us any good we have to be able to put it into action. Our task in Part 2 is to do precisely that - to translate the scientific findings about lowering blood cholesterol through diet into practical, everyday advice about food. This is the "how to" section. Each nutrition guideline developed in Part 1 will be fully explained in terms of foods, not nutrients. The aim is to provide you with all the information you need about what foods to buy, what to cook and how to put meals together. These tools will help you to take control of your cholesterol and manage this problem in the most natural and fundamental way, through food.

10 Key Nutrition Goals of the Pro-Active Plan

Here's a brief summary of the 10 key nutrition goals of the Pro-Active Plan developed in Part 1 and the effects each has on blood cholesterol or other factors affecting heart health. In the pages that follow, we will discuss the food choices needed to achieve these goals.

(1) Increase intake of plant sterols to dramatically lower blood LDL-cholesterol.

(2) Lower intake of saturated fats to lower blood LDL-cholesterol.

(3) Increase intake of plant polyunsaturated fats to lower blood LDL-cholesterol and to increase vitamin E intake.

(4) Lower intake of cholesterol to slightly lower LDL-cholesterol.

(5) Increase intake of marine omega-3 polyunsaturated fats to protect against cardiac arrhythmia (unstable heart beat).

(6) Increase intake of natural antioxidants to help protect LDL-cholesterol against oxidation.

(7) Consume a moderate intake of alcoholic beverages, especially wine, to raise protective HDL-cholesterol levels and to increase antioxidant intake.

(8) Increase dietary quality to increase intake of potentially protective foods and nutrients, to reduce intake of potentially harmful elements of the diet and to help control body weight.

(9) Enjoy a wider variety of foods to ensure nutritional balance.

(10) Enjoy regular physical activity to help control body weight and to raise protective HDL-cholesterol levels.

STEP 1
How do I increase my intake of plant sterols?

Increasing your intake of plant sterols is a particularly important step in reducing your blood cholesterol and one that quickly shows results. Fortunately, increasing your intake of plant sterols is very easy to do. Plant sterols are now incorporated into margarines designed specifically to reduce blood cholesterol. All you need to do is include about 25 grams of plant sterol-enriched spread each day in your meals. Ideally, some plant sterol-enriched spread should be consumed at each meal. However, twice per day with meals is still very effective.

Choose:

> Toast with spread for breakfast.
> A sandwich with spread for lunch.
> A dinner roll with spread with the evening meal.
> Potato or other vegetables with spread.
> Main meals which include spread (see recipes page 127).
> Baked goods made with spread (see recipes page 152).

...include a plant sterol-enriched spread in at least two, preferably three, meals each day...

Benefit
Plant sterols dramatically reduce blood cholesterol by blocking the absorption of cholesterol from the gut.

STEP 2

How do I lower my intake of saturated fats?

Lowering your intake of saturated fat will significantly lower your blood cholesterol. Unfortunately, lowering saturated fat intake does not involve one change in your eating habits, but a great many. Saturated fat is found in a wide range of foods. As a result, lowering saturated fat intake is the most complicated aspect of the Pro-Active Plan. Our main target will be foods containing animal fats, though there are a few vegetable fats we need to be aware of too. We will focus on the three major sources of saturated fats in our diet—dairy products, processed meat and baked goods.

(1) Reduce your intake of dairy fats.

The first of the animal fats to target is dairy fat. Of all the animal fats, dairy fat is the most cholesterol-raising. The less dairy fat you eat the better. This does not mean "give up dairy foods". Rather, include a variety of low-fat dairy foods in your daily meals. These provide most of the valuable nutrients of dairy foods, including calcium, without the damaging saturated fat.

Choose:

Low-fat milks.
Low-fat yoghurts.
Low-fat cheeses (less than 10 per cent fat), in moderation.
Low-fat ice confections, some gelati, sorbet, low-fat frozen yoghurt.

Limit:

Butter - one of the richest sources of saturated fat.
Cheese, reduced-fat cheese.
Cream, sour cream. Ice-cream (full-fat).
Full-fat yoghurt.

...choose low-fat dairy foods...

> **Benefit**
> Lowering saturated fat intake reduces blood cholesterol.

(2) Reduce your intake of fat from meat.

Meat fat is a problem too. About half the fats in meat fat are saturated so it comes as no surprise that meat fat raises blood cholesterol. As a general rule, the less meat fat you eat the better. Again, this does not mean giving up meat. Give up *fatty* meat, especially processed sausage meats. Lean meat is fine and highly recommended. It has many important nutrients to offer.

The goodness of lean meat

Lean meat is low in saturated fat and contains many essential nutrients - high quality protein, iron, zinc, niacin, riboflavin, thiamin and polyunsaturated fatty acids. It's a valuable part of a heart healthy diet.

Choose:

> Lean cuts of red meat.
> Skinless chicken - great in stir-fries.
> Regular meals of fish.
> Polyunsaturated sunflower oil for cooking.

Limit:

> All fatty meats.
> All sausage meats.
> Luncheon meats.
> Processed meat and chicken products.
> Chicken skin.
> Lard, dripping, solid frying fats.

...choose lean meats...

Major sources of saturated fat

The three major sources of saturated fat in out diet are dairy products, processed meats and baked goods.

---

(3) Reduce your intake of fat from commercial baked foods.

Most commercial pastries, cakes and biscuits are rich in saturated fats. They contribute about one fifth of the saturated fats in our diet. There is not an easy replacement for the saturated fat in these foods as it is required to give baked products their form. A biscuit is only crisp because of the hard, saturated fats it contains. Unfortunately, there are not too many commercial baked foods which meet our needs. It is best to limit all these foods. If we want to enjoy some baked foods as a treat, it's best to make some at home using a plant sterol-enriched spread.

Choose:

Home-made biscuits, in moderation (see recipe on page 160).
Home-made cakes, in moderation (see recipe on page 159).
Filo pastry, made with polyunsaturated oil.

Limit:

All commercial biscuits.
All commercial cakes.
All commercial pastries and pies.

...prepare baked goods at home...

What does "reduced-fat" mean on food labels?

Food manufacturers may claim a product is "reduced-fat" if it contains 25 per cent less fat than the standard version. However, this does not necessarily mean the product is low in fat. For example, a standard cheese may contain about 35 per cent dairy fat by weight. The "reduced-fat" version would contain 26 per cent dairy fat - still an exceedingly rich source of saturated fat.

Putting the Pro-Active Plan into Action

(4) Reduce your intake of commercial deep-fried foods, unless they are cooked in a healthy oil.

Most people wouldn't dream of eating foods fried in meat fat at home. Yet we do it all the time when we eat out. Tallow (beef and lamb fat) is one of the most common fats to be found in commercial deep-fryers. Fats based on palm oil are also very popular. Both of these are rich in saturated fats and are cholesterol-raising. Palm oil is one of the few vegetable oils which is rich in saturated fat. It's no better than meat fat.

Fortunately, some shops and clubs are now beginning to use healthier frying fats. These may include cottonseed oil, which is acceptable, or sunflower-based oils which are excellent. What frying fat does your local take-away store use?

"Cholesterol-Free" Vegetable Oils

Beware of oil in take-away shops that claims to be "cholesterol-free" vegetable oil. This claim means little by itself as all vegetable oils are free of cholesterol. However, vegetable oils differ markedly in their saturated fat content. Some "cholesterol free" oils, such as palm oil, are rich in saturated fats and best avoided. Ask the proprietor of the shop whether the oil is approved by the National Heart Foundation.

---

(5) Reduce your intake of fried or baked snack foods, unless they are cooked in a healthy oil.

Like take-aways, most snack foods are fried in meat fat or palm oil - highly saturated fats. This whole category of foods is on our hit list. Don't be fooled by those snack foods that claim to be "baked, not fried". These may contain the same cholesterol-raising fats, in the same amounts as the traditional fried products. The good news is that at least one manufacturer of potato crisps is now frying in sunflower oil and proclaiming it loudly on the label. This is a snack food you can enjoy.

... like palm oil, coconut oil is a vegetable oil, which is high in saturated fats ...

(6) Reduce your intake of fat from confectionary.

Although confectionary usually plays a small role in the diets of adults, there are a few issues we need to be aware of. One of the commonly used fats in confectionary is coconut oil. Like palm oil, coconut oil is a vegetable oil which is high in saturated fats. Processed coconut oil melts in the mouth in a similar way to chocolate and is used in confectionary and baked goods. Many "choc" components of ice-creams and sweets are not chocolate at all, but coconut oil in disguise.

Choose:

> Only those fried take-aways cooked in healthy oils.
> Low-fat foods when eating out.
> Nuts as a snack.
> Snack foods prepared with healthy oils.
> Low-fat confectionary.

Limit:

> Everything out of a commercial deep-fryer, unless cooked in
>   healthy oils.
> All deep-fried snack foods, unless cooked in a healthy oil.
> All baked snack foods, unless prepared with a healthy oil.
> "Choc" confectionary and ice-cream.

Is it true that chocolate doesn't raise cholesterol?

You may have heard that the type of fat in chocolate doesn't raise cholesterol. This depends very much on the type of chocolate in question. One ingredient of all chocolate is cocoa butter which indeed contains fats that have a neutral effect on blood cholesterol. However, different chocolates contain differing amounts of cocoa butter and other ingredients. Milk chocolate obviously contains milk and dairy fat is very cholesterol-raising. Cheap "chocolate" may be little more than flavoured saturated fat.

Putting the Pro-Active Plan into Action

STEP 3

How do I increase my intake of plant polyunsaturated fats?

The polyunsaturated fats in plants lower blood cholesterol. The best source of polyunsaturated fats are vegetable oils such as sunflower, soy bean and safflower oils. Sunflower oil is an excellent choice (see Chapter 3) and has the added benefits of being readily available and cheap. As you would expect, foods which contain sunflower oil such as some margarines, salad dressings and mayonnaise are also excellent sources. Nuts are also useful sources of polyunsaturated fats. Walnuts are especially rich, while Brazils, peanuts and pistachios contain moderate amounts. Wholemeal bread and wholegrain cereals contain polyunsaturated fat too.

Choose:

A plant-sterol enriched spread made with polyunsaturated oils.
Sunflower oil for cooking.
Sunflower oil in salad dressings (see page 124 for ideas).
Nuts as a snack.
Wholemeal bread and wholegrain breakfast cereals.

Limit:

Low-fat spreads.
No-oil salad dressings.

... use sunflower oil in cooking and in salad dressings ...

Benefit
Polyunsaturated oils lower blood cholesterol and are rich in vitamin E.

How can I increase my intake of polyunsaturated fats and lose weight at the same time?

The first thing that many people give up when they attempt to lose weight is anything with any fat in it. However, using low-fat spreads and no-oil dressings to save a few kilojoules is ill-advised. Polyunsaturated fats are too good to give up. They are cholesterol-lowering, essential nutrients and excellent sources of vitamin E. When watching your weight, the key is to cut out the bad, saturated fats (saving yourself some kilojoules) while retaining your intake of polyunsaturated fats.

Putting the Pro-Active Plan into Action ▲

STEP 4
How do I lower my cholesterol intake?

As explained in Chapter 4, the amount of cholesterol in the food we eat has only a small effect on the level of cholesterol in the blood. Plant sterols, saturated fats and polyunsaturated fats have more significant effects. Nevertheless, every little bit helps and keeping your dietary cholesterol intake down is worthwhile, and this is quite easy to do.

As cholesterol is only found in animal foods, we don't need to worry about foods of plant origin such as breads, cereal products, legumes, nuts, fruit, vegetables, vegetable oils and margarines. All of these products are free of cholesterol.

Reducing intake of animal fats to reduce saturated fat also helps to remove a lot of cholesterol from our daily meals. A few high cholesterol foods to keep an eye on include eggs, offal meats and some seafood. Moderation is advised when consuming these foods.

Choose:

Plenty of plant foods.

Limit:

Eggs.
Brains, liver, and kidney.
Prawns, scampi, calamari, squid, octopus.

...eat plenty of plant foods...

Benefit
Reducing intake of cholesterol from food slightly reduces blood cholesterol.

Isn't seafood good for me?

Seafood such as prawns, scampi, calamari, squid and octopus present us with something of a dilemma. On the one hand, they're low in saturated fat and contain beneficial marine omega-3 polyunsaturated fats - both key elements of the Pro-Active Plan. On the other, they're quite high in animal sterols similar to cholesterol - a slight negative. On balance, they're very good foods which can find a place in your meals. Eating them once a week is fine. If you're in the habit of consuming these foods several times a week you may like to pare this back a little and choose more fish.

STEP 5

How do I increase my intake of marine omega-3 polyunsaturated fats?

The special omega-3 polyunsaturated fats found in fish provide unique protection for the heart and promote a normal, steady heart beat. Although the benefit of marine omega-3s is a complicated area of the science of nutrition (see Chapter 7), putting the recommendation into practice is easy. Eat more fish! All fish are highly recommended. However, the best sources of marine omega-3 polyunsaturated fats are the so-called "oily" fish - salmon, sardines, tuna, mackerel and gemfish. These may be enjoyed in fresh or canned form. The canning process does not affect the level of marine polyunsaturated fats and, in fact, helps preserve these rather fragile substances from the ravages of air and light.

Choose:

Two or more fish meals each week.
Plenty of canned fish (see page 162 for ideas).

Limit:

Fish fried in saturated fats.

...eat fish at least twice a week...

Benefit
Oily fish such as salmon and sardines contain marine omega-3 polyunsaturated fats, which provide unique protection against arrhythmia or unstable heart beat.

STEP 6

How do I increase my intake of natural antioxidants?

Natural antioxidants in foods may have important protective roles to play against heart disease (see Chapter 5). Vitamin E appears to be particularly important but may well work in concert with an array of other antioxidants. Some antioxidants, like vitamin E and the carotenoids, are found in the fatty part of foods. Others, like vitamin C and the polyphenols, are found in the watery part of foods. As a result, full antioxidant protection will only be achieved with a combination of both high-fat and low-fat foods. Antioxidant balance may be disrupted if excessive amounts of one antioxidant is consumed, so supplements are not recommended.

Choose:

Sunflower oil for cooking and salads - one of the best sources of vitamin E.

A plant sterol-enriched spread based on sunflower oil for vitamin E.

Plenty of nuts - for vitamin E.

Plenty of vegetables - for vitamin C, carotenoids and some polyphenols.

Plenty of fruit - for vitamin C, carotenoids and some polyphenols.

Tea as preferred hot beverage - the best source of polyphenols.

Limit:

Antioxidant supplements.

...enjoy plenty of nuts, fruits, vegetables and tea...

Benefit
Natural antioxidants help protect LDL-cholesterol from oxidation.

Putting the Pro-Active Plan into Action

STEP 7

What is a moderate intake of alcoholic beverages?

If you're in the habit of drinking alcoholic beverages, there's no reason to give up for the sake of your heart. As we saw in Chapter 6, small quantities of alcohol actually have a protective effect on the heart. However, high intakes of alcohol are not only intoxicating but harmful to many organs of the body. Moderation is the key. Optimal health effects are achieved at two drinks per day for men and one drink per day for women. Wine, beer and other alcoholic drinks appear to offer protection at this level of intake. Red wine may offer another benefit due to its high antioxidant content.

Choose:

> Wine as the preferred alcoholic beverage.
> Up to two drinks per day for men.
> Up to one drink per day for women.

Limit:

> Higher intakes of alcohol.

...enjoy a glass of wine with dinner...

Benefit
Regular intakes of small quantities of red wine increase levels of protective HDL-cholesterol and provide antioxidants.

STEP 8

How do I increase dietary quality?

Improving dietary quality is all about getting nutritional value for money. Some components of our daily meals are more or less valuable than others. For example, foods rich in saturated fat tend to push up blood cholesterol and are obviously poor value for people determined to lower their cholesterol (Chapter 3). If you eat less saturated fat, you improve dietary quality. Sugar is of little value, especially for people watching their weight (Chapter 9). It provides kilojoules but no other nutrients. Dietary quality goes up as sugar intake comes down.

Choices between similar foods can improve dietary quality too. Wholemeal bread and wholegrain cereal products are made from the complete cereal grain, not just part of it. They retain more nutrients and dietary fibre than refined cereal products and white bread. Including some wholegrain cereal products in your daily meals in preference to refined cereals improves dietary quality. Other whole foods include nuts, legumes, vegetables and fresh fruit. Eating plenty of these foods improves dietary quality.

Choose:

Wholemeal bread, in preference to white.
Wholegrain breakfast cereals, in preference to refined cereals.
Plenty of vegetables.
Plenty of fruit.
Plenty of nuts.
Plenty of legumes, including soy.

Limit:

Foods rich in saturated fats.
Foods rich in sugar, especially soft drinks.

...include more wholegrain cereals and less sugar...

Benefit
High dietary quality ensures greater intake of protective nutrients and fewer kilojoules.

STEP 9
How do I eat a wide variety of foods?

Eating a wide variety of foods is one of the fundamental principles of good nutrition. No single food has all the nutrients that adults need to meet their bodies' needs. Different foods contain different nutrients in different amounts. By choosing a variety of foods we get enough of what we need, without an excess of one thing or another. It is all about balance.

Because they are generally low in saturated fat, foods from plant sources are highly recommended for people watching their cholesterol. However, to ensure good nourishment, it's wise to include a wide variety of plant foods. This may entail including new types of foods in your daily meals, perhaps some nuts or soy products. Also, some more variety within foods groups is desirable - different types of nuts, fruits and vegetables. Perhaps you could consider introducing some new foods to your daily meals. How about legumes such as kidney beans and soy beans? Broaden your food horizons.

A variety of low-fat animal foods is recommended. Certainly include some fish. Skinless chicken and different types of lean red meat also have a place.

Choose:

> Different types of vegetables - green, yellow and red.
> A variety of fruits, not just an apple a day.
> Mixed nuts, not just one type.
> Some new plant foods such as soy and other legumes.
> Different types of protein foods - fish, chicken, lean beef and lean pork.

...broaden your food horizons...

Benefit
A wide variety of foods ensures nutritional balance.

STEP 10
What is regular physical activity?

Regular physical activity is not a nutrition goal. Nevertheless it is highly recommended for everyone concerned about cholesterol and heart health and is the key to the long-term control of body weight. It's always a good idea to talk to your doctor before increasing your activity level. Always be guided by his or her opinion.

Regular physical activity means at least 30 minutes of moderate activity most days of the week. For those people unused to activity, this means a considerable increase. The best way to increase physical activity is a personal thing. Some people like to swim; others like to walk. Some like to go-it-alone; others like to join a group. Some people play golf; others like tennis. Take an approach which suits you. Here are a few ideas to help you make your decisions.

▶ Think about your current activity

Consider your current level of physical activity. Are you one of those people who sits to have breakfast, sits in the car on the way to work, sits at a desk all day, sits in the traffic again, sits at the dinner table, sits in front of the TV, then lies in bed for the next eight hours? How much of your day do you spend standing or walking? How often do you walk for 30 minutes at a time? Think about what you are doing now?

▶ Select activities

Consider which activities you would like to engage in. Walking is preferred by most people, but choose what you like. Start slowly, then work up to at least 30 minutes each day. The idea is to get your muscles moving and to lift your heart rate a little.

▶ Identify opportunities for activity

Sift through each day of the week and write down times when you would be able to engage in some activity. Now, review those days when you are "too busy" for some exercise. Make time on these days. Cancel something - increased physical activity has to be a high priority. Any time spent in front of the TV is spare time!

▶ **Schedule your activity**

Write down your planned activity each week - put it in your diary or write it on your calendar. Make physical activity a regular and normal part of your day - part of your routine. If you get bored, find other activities to your liking - the possibilities are endless.

▶ **Review your progress**

Each day, review your progress with physical activity. Did you engage in the exercise you had planned? Do you need to make any adjustments to your daily routine? Eventually you will establish a pattern of physical activity that suits you and your lifestyle. Once this point is reached, stick to it and notice the benefits that flow - you feel lighter on your feet; it's easier to walk up stairs; you have less shortness of breath.

...start slowly - aim for a 30 minute walk each day...

Benefit
Regular physical activity improves fitness, raises blood levels of protective HDL-cholesterol and is essential for long-term weight control.

Let's go shopping!

Now that we have some idea about the type of foods required for the Pro-Active Plan, it's time to do some shopping and stock the larder. Here are some key foods which should be on your shopping list each week.

Key Foods

Plant-sterol enriched spread

Sunflower oil

Fish, canned fish

Lean meat, skinless chicken

Fruit - all types

Vegetables - all types

Nuts - all types

Low-fat milk, low-fat yoghurt

Wholemeal bread, wholegrain breakfast cereal

Tea

Meal Ideas

The variety of tasty meals available on the Pro-Active Plan is as wide as your imagination. Below, the basic principle will be explained with a few examples. However, you'll soon see how flexible the Plan is. There's ample opportunity to modify meals to suit yourself. Remember, including a plant sterol-enriched spread is the single most important decision you need to make at each meal for optimal cholesterol-lowering.

Planning meals has just two steps:

Step 1: Include a plant sterol-enriched spread with your meals.
Make this decision first, then build your meal around it.

Step 2: To complete your meal, include a variety of key foods from Table 1.

TABLE 1

Include several choices with each meal.

Bread, preferably wholemeal.
Wholegrain breakfast cereals, muesli, rolled oats.
Pasta, rice, noodles.
All vegetables—fresh and frozen.
All legumes—soy beans, baked beans.
All herbs.
Vegetable soup.
Vegetable juice.
Tomato-based pasta sauces.
All fruit—fresh, dried and canned .
Fruit juice.
All nuts.
Fresh fish, canned fish.
Lean red meat, skinless chicken.
Low-fat milks.
Low-fat yoghurt.
Tea.
Sunflower oil.
Mayonnaise/salad dressing made with sunflower oil.

Breakfast ideas:

Let's work out a few options for breakfast. First step: choose a way of including a plant sterol spread in your meal, e.g. toast with plant sterol spread. Now select a variety of foods from Table 1. Look at the range of breakfasts available.

Early starter
  *Toast with plant sterol-enriched spread.
  * Fruit low-fat yoghurt.
  * Fruit juice.

Light breakfast
  *Toast with plant sterol-enriched spread.
  * Tinned fruit.
  * Tea.

Hot breakfast
  * Toast with plant sterol-enriched spread.
  * Baked beans with grilled tomato.
  * Porridge with low-fat milk.
  * Tea.

Hearty breakfast
  *Wholewheat cereal with low-fat milk.
  * Sliced banana.
  * Sardines on toast with plant sterol-enriched spread.
  * Tea.

... choose a breakfast that suits your taste and lifestyle ...

Light meal ideas:

Here are some simple, light meals. First step: decide how you're going to include a plant sterol-enriched spread in your meal. How about on a wholemeal bread roll? Now select what you like from Table 1.

Winter warmer
* Bread roll with plant sterol-enriched spread.
* Vegetable soup.
* Fresh fruit.

Summer roll
* Bread roll with plant sterol-enriched spread.
* Tinned salmon.
* Salad vegetables.
* Fresh orange juice.

Salads
* Bread roll with plant sterol-enriched spread.
* Lean chicken.
* Salad (see page 125 for ideas).
* Salad dressing (see page 124 for ideas).
* Fresh fruit.

... vary your meals from day to day ...

Main meal ideas:

Let's get a little adventurous now and plan some main meals - one Mediterranean and one good old favourite. First step - choose a means of including a plant sterol-enriched spread at each meal. Using recipes from the back of this book, build your meals. All the ingredients will be found in Table 1.

Mediterranean feast
* Mediterranean soup (see recipe page 137).
* Italian bread spread with plant sterol-enriched spread.
* Roasted Vegetable Lasagne (see recipe page 141).
* Pumpkin Risotto with Chicken (see recipe page 139).
* Tomato and Basil Salad (see page 125).

Old Favourite
* Veal in Tomato and Onion Gravy (see recipe page 129).
* Mashed potatoes and sweet potato with plant sterol-enriched spread.
* Sugar snap peas.
* Beans.
* Poached pears with low-fat yoghurt.

... enjoy foods from different cuisines ...

Eating out:

When eating out, things are always a little out of your control. Don't worry about it. What you eat at one meal in a week is not going to have a great influence on your blood cholesterol if the other 20 meals have been carefully chosen. And, after all, we usually eat out either to have a little fun or to give the cook in the family a break. The idea is to make the most of the situation.

Firstly, choose your restaurant. If you end up at Greasy Joe's, making a healthy choice is always going to be difficult. An Asian restaurant is a good option - unsaturated vegetable oils are usually used in cooking, the foods are generally low in animal fat and include plenty of vegetables. An Italian restaurant should offer many of the same advantages, though dairy foods will be present.

Choose wisely from the menu. No matter which restaurant you choose, there will always be some choices on the menu which are better than others for people who are watching their cholesterol. If you're in doubt about any menu item, ask about it. Don't be afraid to ask staff in restaurants about their foods. It makes them think about their customers' expectations.

Finally, enjoy your meal. Enjoying good food around the table with family or friends is one of life's great pleasures.

Recipes

If you really love food you probably love to cook. This is the section for you. It contains a variety of tasty recipes and ideas suitable for all eating occasions. Lowering your cholesterol never tasted so good! Each recipe and idea has been developed using the key ingredients of the Pro-Active Plan and has been thoroughly tested.

Taking the latest nutrition findings and translating them into good-tasting, easy to prepare meals needed the guiding hand of an expert. Experienced food editor, Veronica Cuskelly, rose to the challenge. Veronica's own words sum up the gastronomic treats that appear on the pages that follow:

"These recipes show there is no need to compromise on flavour when preparing meals for the Pro-Active Plan. There is plenty of scope for classic favourites, some examples of modern cuisine and even a few indulgences. Ample choice is available to meet personal or family needs. These recipes are simple to prepare and most important of all, delicious."

10 Suggested Spread Ideas

Hot and Tasty Breads

Preparation Time: 10-15 minutes
Cooking Time: 25-30 minutes

125g (¹/₂ cup) Flora pro-activ spread

Flavouring (see chart)

1 large or 2 small French bread sticks

1. Mix Flora pro-activ spread and flavouring of choice until well combined.
2. Slice bread stick/s into 1cm slices. Spread each side of the bread with flavoured spread, reshape stick/s, wrap in foil and bake at 180°C for 25-30 minutes, unwrapping the foil during the last 5 minutes of cooking.
3. Serve with soups, main meals and at barbecues.

Serves 8-10.

> **Hint:** Leftover spread may be wrapped in plastic wrap and kept in the refrigerator for up to three days.

Tips:
* Spread on sandwiches, breads or crispbread.
* Stir through cooked pasta.
* Toss through cooked vegetables.

FLAVOURED SPREADS

	VARIETY	ADD
1.	Garlic	2-3 crushed garlic cloves
2.	Herb and Garlic	2 tablespoons chopped fresh parsley and 2 crushed garlic cloves
3.	Apricot and Almond	$1/4$ cup chopped dried apricots and $1/4$ cup chopped roasted almonds
4.	Roasted Walnut	$1/2$ cup chopped roasted walnuts
5.	Roasted Capsicum	2 tablespoons finely chopped roasted capsicum
6.	Sun-dried Tomato	2 tablespoons finely chopped sun-dried tomatoes
7.	Onion and Rosemary	2 tablespoons finely chopped onion and 1 teaspoon finely chopped fresh rosemary
8.	Herb	1 teaspoon finely chopped fresh sage, oregano and $1/2$ teaspoon thyme leaves
9.	Olive	2 tablespoons finely chopped black olives
10.	Pizza	2 teaspoons tomato paste, I crushed garlic clove, 2 finely chopped anchovies

10 Salad Ideas

Salad Dressings

Basic dressing

Preparation Time: 5 minutes

> **165mL (²/₃ cup) sunflower oil**
>
> **60mL (¹/₄ cup) white or red wine vinegar**
>
> **¹/₂ - 1 teaspoon Dijon mustard**
>
> **1 teaspoon caster sugar**
>
> **Salt and pepper, optional**

1. Place oil, vinegar, mustard and sugar in a bowl and, using a wire whisk, mix until the sugar has dissolved.

2. Taste dressing and season with salt and pepper.

3. Store in the refrigerator in a screwtop jar. Use as required.

Makes approximately 1 cup.

FLAVOURED DRESSINGS

ITALIAN	Use balsamic vinegar, grain mustard and add 1 tablespoon each chopped fresh parsley and fresh oregano and 1 teaspoon chopped fresh marjoram.
HERB	Add 1 tablespoon each chopped fresh chives and fresh sage and 1 teaspoon chopped fresh thyme.
ASIAN	Substitute the vinegar with 1 tablespoon soy sauce and the Dijon mustard with 1 teaspoon grated ginger or sweet chilli sauce.

SALADS		DRESSING
1.	Mixed Lettuce and Baby Spinach	Basic / Italian / Herb
2.	Mesclun, Roma Tomatoes, Spanish Onion	Basic / Italian / Herb
3.	Mushroom, Shallot and Walnut	Basic / Italian / Herb
4.	Tomato and Basil	Basic / Italian
5.	Asparagus, Red Capsicum and Toasted Almond	Italian / Herb
6.	Prawn, Pineapple and Mignonette Lettuce	Basic
7.	Rare Roast Beef, Coriander, Cherry Tomato and Lettuce	Asian
8.	Cooked Chicken, Cos Lettuce, Yellow Capsicum and Croutons	Basic / Italian / Herb
9.	Chinese Cabbage, Carrot and Chives	Asian
10.	Cooked New Potatoes, Shallots and Mint	Herb

Suggestions

Enjoy a salad as a starter or main course.

Serve as side salads with grills, cold cuts and barbecues.

Use as fillings for pocket breads, sandwiches and rolls.

10 Sandwich Ideas

Traditional and Open Sandwiches

Preparation Time: 10 minutes

5-10g (1-2 teaspoons) Flora pro-activ

1 or 2 slices of bread of choice

Filling or topping of choice (see chart)

1. Spread each slice of bread with Flora pro-activ.
2. Top with filling.
3. Serve as an open sandwich or top with another spread slice of bread.

Makes 1 sandwich.

SANDWICH TOPPINGS OR FILLINGS

1.	Ham, Lettuce and Mustard
2.	Shaved Chicken with Mango Chutney
3.	Roast Beef, Tomato and Pickle
4.	Shaved Turkey, Alfalfa Sprouts and Cranberry Sauce
5.	Salmon, Capers and Dill
6.	Sardine and Onion
7.	Tuna, Lettuce and Tomato
8.	Avocado and Sweet Chilli
9.	Lamb, Mint Sauce and Baby Spinach
10.	Carrot, Sultanas and Walnuts

10 Classic Favourites

Chicken and Corn Soup

Preparation Time: 15 minutes
Cooking Time: 35 minutes

20mL (1 tablespoon) sunflower oil

1 onion, finely chopped

2 cups fresh corn kernels or 1 x 400g can corn kernels, drained

750mL (3 cups) chicken stock

300g chicken breast fillet, finely diced

Salt and pepper, optional

¹/₄ cup finely chopped shallots

1. Heat oil in a saucepan over a low heat and cook onion for 2-3 minutes or until soft. Stir in the corn and stock and bring to the boil. Cover and cook for 15-20 minutes, stirring occasionally. Remove from heat.
2. Blend or process until almost smooth. Return to heat, stir in the chicken, cover and cook for a further 3-5 minutes or until the chicken is thoroughly cooked. Season to taste with salt and pepper.
3. Serve sprinkled with shallots accompanied by Apricot and Almond Bread (see recipe page 123) or crusty bread spread with Flora pro-activ.

Serves 4.

Chunky Vegetable Soup

Preparation Time: 15 minutes
Cooking Time: 40 minutes

¹/₄ cup pearl barley

185mL (³/₄ cup) water

20mL (1 tablespoon) sunflower oil

1 small onion, chopped

1 medium carrot, diced

1 small parsnip, diced

¹/₂ swede, diced

1 zucchini, diced

1 x 500g jar pasta sauce

750mL (3 cups) water

1 bay leaf

Salt and pepper, optional

¹/₄ cup finely chopped fresh parsley

1. Place barley and water in a saucepan, bring to the boil, reduce heat, cover and cook for 35 minutes or until tender.

2. In the meantime, heat oil in a large saucepan over a low heat, add onion and cook for 3-5 minutes, stirring occasionally. Add vegetables and, stirring occasionally, cook for 5 minutes. Stir in the pasta sauce, water and bay leaf, cover and simmer for 20 minutes or until the vegetables are tender. Remove bay leaf. Add barley and water and reheat. Season to taste.

3. Serve sprinkled with parsley accompanied by Herb Bread (see recipe page 123) or crusty bread spread with Flora pro-activ.

Serves 4 as a main meal.

Veal in Tomato and Onion Gravy

Preparation Time: 10 minutes
Cooking Time: 25 minutes

1 ¹/₂ tablespoons flour

Salt and pepper, optional

500g (8 small steaks) veal rump, trimmed

40mL (2 tablespoons) sunflower oil

1 medium onion, thinly sliced

20mL (1 tablespoon) sweet sherry

3 medium tomatoes, sliced

165mL (²/₃ cup) beef stock

1. Place flour, salt and pepper in a plastic bag. Add steaks, in batches, and shake to coat.
2. Heat half the oil in a large frying pan, add veal and cook on each side, 3-4 minutes or until thoroughly cooked. Remove and set aside.
3. Heat remaining oil in pan, add onion and cook until soft. Add sherry and stir until evaporated. Stir in the tomatoes and stock and cook for 5 minutes. Return veal to pan, simmer for 5 minutes. Serve with Mashed Potatoes. (see recipe page 149), steamed sugar snap peas and beans.

Serves 4.

Roast Lamb with Rosemary and Creamed Roasted Garlic

Preparation Time: 10 minutes
Cooking Time: 1 hour + 20-30 minutes resting time

1.5kg leg lamb

10 sprigs rosemary

4 heads garlic

10mL (2 teaspoons) sunflower oil

5g (1 teaspoon) Flora pro-activ

1. Pre-heat oven to 210°C.

2. Using a sharp knife, make 10 slits in lamb and insert sprigs of rosemary. Place lamb on a rack in a baking dish and bake for 10 minutes. In the meantime, brush garlic heads with oil and wrap each one in foil. Reduce oven temperature to 180°C and place garlic on rack. Bake with lamb for 45 minutes or until lamb is cooked and garlic is soft. Wrap lamb in foil and rest for 20-30 minutes. Cut tops off garlic heads and squeeze the cloves into a bowl. Cream garlic with Flora pro-activ.

3. Serve lamb sliced with Roast Vegetables (see recipe page 147) and Creamed Roasted Garlic.

Note: Lamb should be eaten with all visible fat trimmed.

Serves 6.

Chicken and Vegetable Curry

Preparation Time: 20 minutes
Cooking Time: 30 minutes

40mL (2 tablespoons) sunflower oil

$1/2$ cup finely chopped onion

1 garlic clove, crushed

2 tablespoons mild curry powder

1 tablespoon plain flour

1 $1/2$ cups chopped carrot

1 $1/2$ cups cubed potato

1 $1/4$ cups chicken stock

500g cubed chicken breast fillet

1 cup frozen peas

Salt and pepper, optional

1. Heat oil in a saucepan over a low heat, add the onion and cook for 2-3 minutes. Add the garlic, curry powder and flour and continue cooking, stirring constantly, for a further 2-3 minutes.
2. Add the carrot, potato and stock and bring to the boil. Cover and cook, stirring occasionally, for 10-12 minutes or until the vegetables are just cooked. Add the chicken and, continuing to stir, cook for a further 6 minutes. Stir in the peas, cook for a further 2 minutes or until the chicken is thoroughly cooked.
3. Season with salt and pepper to taste and serve with rice.

Serves 4.

Beef Casserole

Preparation Time: 15 minutes
Cooking Time: 1 ¹/₂ hours

2 tablespoons plain flour

500g gravy beef, trimmed and thinly sliced

40mL (2 tablespoons) sunflower oil

3 tomatoes, sliced

2 onions, sliced

1 potato, sliced

1 carrot, sliced

250mL (1 cup) beef stock

1. Pre-heat oven to 160°C.

2. Place flour in a plastic bag. Add beef, in batches, and shake to coat. Heat oil in a frying pan and brown beef in batches, set aside. Layer meat, tomato, onions, potatoes and carrots in a 1.5-litre casserole dish. Pour over the stock, cover and bake for 1 ¹/₂ hours or until cooked.

3. Serve with peas or beans, crusty bread spread with Flora pro-activ or Garlic Bread (see recipe page 123)

Serves 4.

Tuna and Carrot Pasta Bake

Preparation Time: 20 minutes
Baking Time: 20 minutes

2 cups pasta, penne or bows

1 $1/2$ cups sliced carrot

60g ($1/4$ cup) Flora pro-activ

30g (1 $1/2$ tablespoons) plain flour

2 teaspoons wholegrain mustard

625mL (2 $1/2$ cups) reduced-fat milk

$1/4$ cup chopped fresh parsley

1 x 425g can tuna, drained

$1/2$ cup dry breadcrumbs

$1/4$ cup slivered almonds

20g (1 tablespoon) Flora pro-activ, extra

1. Pre-heat oven to 190°C. Brush a 2-litre capacity dish with Flora pro-activ. Cook pasta according to pack directions, drain.
2. Place carrot in a saucepan with a little water, cover and cook over a low heat for 6-8 minutes, stirring occasionally. Drain carrot and set aside.
3. Place Flora pro-activ, flour and mustard into the saucepan and, stirring constantly, cook for 1-2 minutes. Gradually whisk in the milk and cook until the sauce comes to the boil. Continue whisking and cook for 2-3 minutes. Remove from heat and stir in the parsley, tuna, pasta and carrot. Place mixture into prepared dish. Combine breadcrumbs, almonds and extra Flora pro-activ and sprinkle over the mixture. Bake for 20 minutes or until golden. Serve with Mesclun, Roma Tomatoes and Spanish Onion Salad (see recipe page 125).

Serves 4-6.

Recipes

133

Smoked Cod with Onion and Parsley Sauce

Preparation Time: 10 minutes
Cooking Time: 20 minutes

375mL (1 ¹/₂ cups) water

250mL (1 cup) low-fat milk

4 x 150g smoked cod fillets

60g (¹/₄ cup) Flora pro-activ

1 onion, finely chopped

1 ¹/₂ tablespoons plain flour

500mL (2 cups) low-fat milk, extra

Salt and pepper, optional

¹/₄ cup finely chopped fresh parsley

1. Place water and milk in a large frying pan, cover and bring to the boil, reduce heat to a simmer. Add cod, skin-side down, cover, and cook for 12-15 minutes of until fish flakes easily, remove, draining well and keep warm.

2. In the meantime, place Flora pro-activ, onion and flour in a saucepan over a low heat and cook, stirring constantly, for 3-5 minutes or until the onion is soft.

3. Gradually add the extra milk and, stirring constantly, cook until the sauce comes to the boil. Continue stirring and cook for 2-3 minutes. Season sauce to taste and stir in the parsley. Serve with the cod, Mashed Potatoes (see recipe page 149) and peas.

Serves 4.

Pan-fried Fish Fillets

Preparation Time: 5 minutes
Cooking Time: 12 minutes

4 x 150g white boneless fish fillets

2 tablespoons plain flour

Salt and pepper, optional

40mL (2 tablespoons) sunflower oil

1. Dry fish fillets with paper towels of excess moisture. Place flour, salt and pepper in a plastic bag. Add fish fillets, in batches, and shake to coat.
2. Heat oil in a frying pan (see Hint), add fish and cook on each side for 3-4 minutes or until golden and flesh flakes easily.
3. Serve with a Mixed Lettuce and Baby Spinach Salad with Herb Dressing (see page 125) and lemon wedges.

Serves 4.

> **Hint:** To test if oil is ready, place the handle of a wooden spoon in the oil and if the oil bubbles around the handle, oil has reached the correct temperature.

Beef Stew with Herb Dumplings

Preparation Time: 15 minutes
Cooking Time: 2 hours

40mL (2 tablespoons) sunflower oil

500g topside steak, trimmed and cubed

1 onion, finely chopped

1 carrot, chopped

1 bay leaf

250mL (1 cup) beef stock

125mL ($^1/_2$ cup) water

1 $^1/_2$ cups plain flour

1 $^1/_2$ teaspoons baking powder

2 teaspoons salt

40g (2 tablespoons) Flora pro-activ

2 tablespoons finely chopped fresh parsley

125-165mL ($^1/_2$ - $^2/_3$ cup) low-fat milk

1 tablespoon plain flour, extra

1. Heat oil in a saucepan, brown meat in batches, set aside.
Add onion and carrot and, stirring, cook for 3-5 minutes. Add meat,
bay leaf, stock and water; bring to the boil. Reduce heat, cover, and
simmer for 1 $^1/_2$ hours or until meat is tender.
2. Sift flour, baking powder and salt in a bowl and, using your
fingertips, rub in Flora pro-activ until mixture resembles fine
breadcrumbs. Using a round-bladed knife, stir in parsley and
sufficient milk until mixture forms a ball. Divide mixture into six
portions and toss in extra flour. Drop dumplings onto simmering
stew, cover and cook for 15 minutes.
3. Serve with steamed snow peas or baby squash.

Serves 4.

10 Modern Favourites

Mediterranean Soup

Preparation Time: 15 minutes
Cooking Time: 30 minutes

20mL (1 tablespoon) sunflower oil

1 onion, finely chopped

1 red capsicum, diced

2 stalks celery, chopped

1 zucchini, chopped

¼ cauliflower, cut into florets

1 litre (4 cups) water

2 teaspoons vegetable stock powder

600mL bottle tomato cooking sauce

300g can butter beans, drained and rinsed

Salt and pepper, optional

Finely chopped fresh basil

1. Heat oil in a large saucepan, add onion, capsicum and celery; cook until onion is soft. Add zucchini, cauliflower, water, stock powder and tomato sauce and stirring occasionally, bring to the boil.
2. Reduce heat, cover and cook, stirring occasionally, for 15 minutes. Stir in beans and reheat. Season to taste.
3. Serve sprinkled with basil, accompanied by Olive Bread (see recipe page 123).

Serves 4.

Asian Beef Noodle Soup

Preparation Time: 15 minutes
Cooking Time: 25 minutes

150g rice noodles

1 bunch bok choy, trimmed, cut into bite-size pieces

10mL (2 teaspoons) sunflower oil

1 small onion, finely chopped

2 medium carrots, sliced

1.5 litres (6 cups) beef stock

1 teaspoon brown sugar

300g beef fillet, cut into thin strips

$1/2$ cup thinly sliced shallots

$1/3$ cup fresh coriander leaves

$1/4$ cup fresh mint leaves, sliced

1 lime, quartered

1. Cook rice noodles according to pack directions. Set aside. Rinse bok choy in water until thoroughly clean. Drain and set aside.
2. Heat oil in a saucepan over a low heat, add onion and cook, stirring occasionally, until soft. Add carrots, stock and sugar, bring to the boil, reduce heat, cover and simmer for 8-10 minutes or until carrot is tender. Add beef, cook for 1 minute or until cooked. Spoon beef and carrots into serving bowls and add noodles.
3. Bring stock back to boil, add bok choy, cover and cook for 3-4 minutes or until tender. Spoon into bowls and garnish with shallots, coriander and mint. Add lime juice to taste. Serve immediately.

Serves 4.

Pumpkin Risotto with Chicken

Preparation Time: 15 minutes
Cooking Time: 45 minutes

1.5 litres (6 cups) chicken or vegetable stock

15-20 saffron threads or $^1/_2$ teaspoon turmeric

20mL (1 tablespoon) sunflower oil

1 garlic clove, crushed

1 large onion, finely chopped

800g pumpkin, cut into 1.5cm cubes

1 $^1/_2$ cups arborio rice

10mL (2 teaspoons) sunflower oil, extra

20g (1 tablespoon) Flora pro-activ

Salt and pepper to taste, optional

500g (4) chicken breast fillets, trimmed

1-2 tablespoons finely chopped fresh parsley

1. Place stock and saffron in a saucepan and bring to the boil.
Reduce heat and continue simmering.
2. Heat oil in a large saucepan, add garlic, onion, pumpkin and rice,
stir, about 4-5 minutes. Add $^1/_3$ cup of simmering stock and continue
to stir over a low heat until stock is absorbed. Add the remaining
stock, in small quantities, stirring constantly until the stock is
absorbed, approximately 30 minutes or until the rice is creamy. (Use
extra boiling water if necessary.) Stir in pro-activ and season to taste.
3. In the meantime, heat extra oil in a non-stick frying pan and
pan-fry chicken until thoroughly cooked. Serve chicken sprinkled with
parsley and accompanied by risotto and an Asparagus, Red Capsicum
and Toasted Almond Salad with Herb Dressing (see page 125).

Serves 4.

Moroccan Lamb with Prunes, Almonds and Couscous

Preparation Time: 15 minutes
Cooking Time: 1 hour

40mL (2 tablespoons) sunflower oil

$1/2$ cup blanched almonds

1kg lamb, trimmed and cubed

2 garlic cloves, crushed

1 large onion, finely chopped

1 cinnamon stick

2 teaspoons ground cumin

$3/4$ teaspoon ground coriander

$1/4$ teaspoon paprika

250g pitted prunes

500mL (2 cups) water

1 $1/2$ cups couscous

310mL (1 $1/4$ cups) boiling vegetable stock

10g (2 teaspoons) Flora pro-activ

1. Heat oil in a saucepan, add the almonds and stir until golden, remove and set aside.

2. Add lamb to the saucepan and brown in batches. Return lamb to the saucepan with garlic, onion, cinnamon, cumin, coriander and paprika and cook for 1 minute. Add the prunes and water and bring to the boil. Cover and simmer for 50 minutes or until the lamb is tender, stirring occasionally.

3. Place couscous in a bowl, stir in boiling stock until liquid is absorbed. Mix in the pro-activ. Serve with lamb, sprinkled with almonds and accompanied by steamed carrot, asparagus and zucchini tossed with Orange and Chive Sauce (see recipe page 150).

Serves 4.

Roasted Vegetable Lasagne

Preparation Time: 30 minutes

Cooking Time: 35 minutes + 15 minutes standing time

Flora pro-activ, melted, for brushing dish

4 medium yellow or green zucchinis, sliced lengthwise

1 large eggplant, sliced lengthwise

4-5 large flat mushrooms

1 large red capsicum, sliced lengthwise

60mL ($1/4$ cup) sunflower oil

737g jar tomato pasta sauce

1 teaspoon sugar

6 instant lasagne sheets

1. Pre-heat oven to 180°C. Brush a 2 $1/2$ - 3-litre capacity dish with melted Flora pro-activ.

2. Heat a char-grill and brush zucchinis, eggplant, mushrooms and capsicum with oil and char-grill. Remove blackened skin from capsicum and slice flesh. Place vegetables on baking trays and bake for 10-12 minutes, cool. Spread a small amount of combined pasta sauce and sugar into prepared dish and line with two lasagne sheets. Layer with zucchinis, pasta sauce, lasagne sheets, eggplant, sauce, lasagne sheets, mushrooms, sauce and finishing with capsicum.

3. Bake for 35 minutes or until cooked. Stand for 15 minutes before serving accompanied by lettuce and Mushroom, Shallot and Walnut Salad with Italian Dressing (see page 125).

Serves 6.

Honey Teriyaki Chicken and Vegetable Stir-fry

Preparation Time: 15 minutes + 30 minutes marinating time
Cooking Time: 15 minutes

500g chicken breast fillet, cut into strips

60mL ($^1/_4$ cup) teriyaki sauce

1 $^1/_2$ tablespoons honey

1 garlic clove, crushed

40mL (2 tablespoons) sunflower oil

4 cups sliced vegetables (broccoli, yellow squash, celery, onion)

1 tablespoon cornflour

$^1/_3$ cup water

1. Place chicken, teriyaki sauce, honey and garlic in a bowl and mix thoroughly. Cover and marinate in the refrigerator for 20-30 minutes. Drain and reserve marinade.
2. Heat a wok over a medium heat and add half the oil. When hot add the vegetables and stir-fry for 3 minutes, then set aside.
3. Add the remaining oil to the wok, add chicken and stir-fry for 3 minutes. Return the vegetables to the wok and stir-fry with chicken for 2-3 minutes or until cooked. Blend the cornflour, water and reserved marinade, add to the chicken and vegetables and bring to the boil. Continue stir-frying for a further 1-2 minutes.
Serve with rice.

Serves 4.

Stir-fry Asian Beef Noodles

Preparation Time: 10 minutes + 30 minutes marinating
Cooking Time: 5 minutes

500g rump steak, trimmed and cut into strips

1 garlic clove, crushed

$1/3$ cup plum sauce

2 tablespoons soy sauce

600g hokkein noodles

40mL (2 tablespoons) sunflower oil

1 large onion, cut into wedges

1 $1/2$ cups sliced beans

165mL ($2/3$ cup) beef stock

1 tablespoon cornflour

1. Place rump strips, garlic, plum sauce and soy sauce into a bowl and mix thoroughly. Cover and marinate in the refrigerator for 20-30 minutes. Drain and reserve marinade.
2. In the meantime, place noodles in a bowl and cover with hot water and mix to separate. Drain and cut roughly.
3. Heat a wok over a medium heat and add half the oil. Add onion and beans and stir-fry for 3 minutes, set aside. Heat remaining oil in the wok, add the beef and stir-fry for 2-3 minutes or until cooked. Return the vegetables to the wok. Mix together the reserved marinade, stock and cornflour and add to the wok. Stir until the sauce comes to the boil. Add the noodles and stir until hot. Serve immediately.

Serves 4.

Sun-dried Tomato and Salmon Cutlet Parcels

Preparation Time: 10 minutes
Cooking Time: 15-20 minutes

4 x 150g salmon cutlets

40g (2 tablespoons) Flora pro-activ Sun-dried Tomato Spread

(see recipe page 123)

1. Pre-heat oven to 180°C.
2. Place each cutlet on a piece of foil and top with 2 teaspoons Sun-dried Tomato Spread. Wrap in parcels and place on a baking slide. Bake for 15-20 minutes or until fish flakes easily.
3. Serve with Roasted Garlic Mashed Potato (see recipe page 149) and steamed asparagus and sugar snap peas.

Serves 4.

Marinated Lamb Cutlets

Preparation Time: 15 minutes + 20 minutes or overnight marinating
Cooking Time: 10 minutes + 10 minutes resting

Zest and juice of 1 lemon

2 teaspoons finely chopped fresh rosemary

20mL (1 tablespoon) sunflower oil

Salt and pepper, optional

12 lamb cutlets, trimmed

1. Combine lemon zest and juice, rosemary, oil, salt and pepper in a bowl and mix well.
2. Place cutlets in one layer in a dish and coat well with the marinade. Cover and refrigerate 20 minutes or overnight.
3. Pre-heat oven to 200°C. Line a baking tray with baking paper and place cutlets on top. Bake cutlets for 10 minutes. Cover with foil and rest for 5-10 minutes. Serve cutlets with Mashed Potato and Sweet Potato (see recipe page 149) and peas.

Serves 4-6.

Hint: Cutlets may also be grilled or pan-fried.

Creamy Mushrooms with Fettuccine

Preparation Time: 15 minutes
Cooking Time: 20 minutes

375g fettuccine

20g (1 tablespoon) Flora pro-activ

1 garlic clove, crushed

1 medium onion, finely chopped

200g button mushrooms, sliced

150g large flat mushrooms, sliced

20g (1 tablespoon) Flora pro-activ, extra

2 tablespoons plain flour

1 teaspoon Dijon mustard

500mL (2 cups) vegetable stock

125mL ($^{1}/_{2}$ cup) low-fat milk

Salt and pepper to taste

1 bunch chives, snipped

1. Cook fettuccine according to pack directions. Drain and set aside.

2. Place Flora pro-activ, garlic and onion in a saucepan and cook over a gentle heat until onion is soft. Add mushrooms and, stirring occasionally, cook for 4-5 minutes. Set aside.

3. Place extra Flora pro-activ, flour and mustard in the saucepan and cook over a gentle heat, stirring constantly, for 2-3 minutes. Gradually add stock and milk, stir until boiling. Reduce heat and cook for a further 2-3 minutes. Stir in the mushroom mixture, reheat and season to taste. Stir in the fettuccine. Serve sprinkled with chives accompanied by Tomato and Basil Salad with Basic Dressing (see page 125).

Serves 4.

Vegetables

Roast Vegetables

Preparation Time: 15 minutes
Cooking Time: 1 hour

3-4 vegetables per person (see chart), sliced

40mL (2 tablespoons) sunflower oil

1. Pre-heat oven to 190°C.
2. Choose 3 or 4 vegetables from the chart below, peel, wash and dry thoroughly.
3. Place oil in a baking dish and heat in the oven. When the oil is hot, carefully add the vegetables and brush each with oil.
Bake for 45-50 minutes, turning once, or until vegetables are golden and tender.

Serves 4.

SUGGESTED VEGETABLES

Carrot
Choko
Onion
Parsnip
Potato
Pumpkin
Sweet potato
Tomatoes

Basic Stir-fried Vegetables

Preparation Time: 10 minutes
Cooking Time: 10 minutes

20mL (1 tablespoon) sunflower oil

3-4 vegetables per person (see chart), sliced

1 garlic clove, crushed

Flavourings of choice (see chart)

1. Peel and wash vegetables.
2. Heat a wok, over high heat, add oil. When the oil is hot, add the vegetables and garlic and flavouring of your choice. Stir-fry until vegetables are just cooked.
3. Serve with rice and/or as an accompaniment to pan-fried or grilled meats.

Serves 4.

SUGGESTED VEGETABLES

Beans
Broccoli
Carrot
Celery
Mushrooms
Onion
Red or Green capsicum
Snow peas
Squash
Zucchinis

FLAVOURINGS	ADD
Thai-style	$1/4$ cup basil leaves, $1/4$ cup coriander leaves and 1 tablespoon grated ginger.
Chinese-style	1-2 tablespoons oyster sauce, 1 tablespoon soy sauce, 1 teaspoon grated ginger.
Indian-style	1-2 teaspoons ground cumin, $1/2$ teaspoon ground turmeric, 1 teaspoon black mustard seeds, 1 garlic clove crushed, 1-2 tablespoons water and serve with a dollop of whipped yoghurt.
Honey Soy	2 tablespoons honey and 1 tablespoon soy sauce.
Sweet Chilli, Lime and Cracked Pepper	1-2 tablespoons sweet chilli sauce, 2 teaspoons cracked pepper and 1 tablespoon lime juice.

Mashed Potatoes

Preparation Time: 10 minutes
Cooking Time: 20-30 minutes

500-600g potatoes + variation choice (see chart)

60g ('/4 cup) Flora pro-activ

85mL ('/3 cup) low-fat milk

Salt and pepper, optional

2 tablespoons finely chopped fresh parsley, optional

1. Peel, wash and cut potatoes and variation of your choice into large cubes.
2. Place in a saucepan and cover with cold water and bring to the boil. Reduce heat and cover and cook until tender. Drain well and mash. Add Flora pro-activ and mix well. Heat milk add to mash and mix until smooth. Stir in the parsley.
3. Serve with cooked meats and fish, casseroles and stews.

Serves 4.

VARIATION	ADD
Potato and Parsnip	200g parsnips and reduce potato to 400g
Potato and Sweet Potato	300g sweet potato and reduce potato to 400g
Potato, Pumpkin and Bacon	300g pumpkin and reduce potato to 400g. Top with crispy bacon.
Potato, Onion and Chive	Before serving add 1 finely chopped onion and 1 tablespoon chopped fresh chives.
Roasted Garlic	Before serving add cloves of 1 head of roasted garlic (see recipe page 130)

Steamed Vegetables

Preparation Time: 10 minutes
Cooking Time: 5-10 minutes

3-4 vegetables per person (see chart)

20g (1 tablespoon) Flora pro-activ

Flavouring of choice (see chart)

SUGGESTED VEGETABLES

Asparagus
Beans
Broccoli
Carrot
Cauliflower
Celery
Pumpkin
Peas
Shallots
Zucchini

1. Peel and wash vegetables. Place vegetables in a steamer over simmering water. Cover and steam for 5-10 minutes or until vegetables are tender.

2. Remove from steamer and place in a bowl. Mix through flavouring of your choice.

3. Serve with grilled, steamed or barbecued meats and fish.

Serves 4.

FLAVOUR	TOSS
Sun-dried Tomato	With 2 tablespoons Sun-dried Tomato Spread (see recipe page 123).
Honey Sesame	With $1/2$-1 tablespoon honey and 1 tablespoon toasted sesame seeds.
Olive and Pine Nuts	With $1/4$ cup sliced black olives and 2 tablespoons toasted pine nuts.
Herb	With $1/4$ cup chopped fresh parsley and 1 teaspoon fresh thyme.
Orange and Chive	With juice of 1 orange and 2-3 tablespoons chopped fresh chives.

10 Great Sauces

Basic White Sauce

40g (2 tablespoons) Flora pro-activ

2 tablespoons flour

500mL (2 cups) reduced-fat milk

1. Place Flora pro-activ and flour in a saucepan and, stirring constantly, cook for 1-2 minutes.
2. Gradually whisk in the milk and cook until the sauce comes to the boil. Continue whisking and cook for 2-3 minutes.
3. Add Flavourings of choice (see chart), reheat and serve with pasta, rice or vegetables.

Serves 4.

FLAVOUR	ADD
Tuna and Parsley	1 x 425g can drained tuna and 1 tablespoon finely chopped fresh parsley.
Salmon and Shallot	1 x 210g can drained salmon and $1/4$ cup chopped shallots.
Ham and Mushroom	125g shaved ham and 2 cups sliced mushrooms.
Chicken and Creamed Corn	25g shaved chicken and 1 x 210g can creamed corn.
Asparagus and Capsicum	1 bunch sliced, cooked asparagus and $1/4$ cup finely diced red capsicum.
Roasted Vegetable and Pine Nuts	250g chopped roasted vegetables (capsicum, eggplant, zucchini) and 1 tablespoon toasted pine nuts.
Olive and Caper	$1/2$ cup sliced, pitted black olives and 1 tablespoon capers.
Dijon Mustard, Honey and Walnut	2 teaspoons Dijon mustard, 1 tablespoon honey and $1/4$ cup chopped walnuts.
Sun-dried Tomato	125g sun-dried tomatoes processed.
Herbed Lemon	1 teaspoon fresh lemon thyme leaves, $1/2$ teaspoon finely chopped fresh oregano and grated rind of 1 lemon.

10 Wonderful Things to Bake

Herb Scones

Preparation Time: 15 minutes
Cooking Time: 15 minutes

2 cups self-raising flour

1 teaspoon baking powder

60g ($^1/_4$ cup) Flora pro-activ

1 tablespoon sugar

1 tablespoon finely chopped fresh parsley

1 tablespoon finely chopped fresh chives

1 teaspoon finely chopped fresh rosemary

1 egg, lightly beaten

$^1/_2$ cup reduced-fat milk

Extra milk for glazing

1. Pre-heat oven to 210°C and line a baking slide with baking paper.
2. Sift flour and baking powder into a bowl. Using your fingertips,
rub in Flora pro-activ until mixture resembles fine breadcrumbs.
Stir in the sugar, parsley, chives and rosemary. Using a round-bladed
knife, stir in egg and milk. Mix until mixture forms a ball.
Toss mixture onto a lightly floured board and knead until smooth.
3. Roll mixture to 15mm thickness and using a scone cutter, cut into
rounds. Place scones close together on prepared baking slide and
brush tops with milk. Bake for 15 minutes or until the scones sound
hollow when tapped. Serve spread with Flora pro-activ.

Makes 12-15.

Date Scones

Preparation Time: 15 minutes
Cooking Time: 15 minutes

2 cups self-raising flour

1 teaspoon baking powder

60g ($^1/_4$ cup) Flora pro-activ

1 tablespoon brown sugar

$^1/_2$ cup chopped dates

$^1/_2$ cup reduced-fat milk

Extra milk for glazing

1. Pre-heat oven to 210°C and line a baking slide with baking paper.
2. Sift flour and baking powder into a bowl. Using your fingertips, rub in Pro-activ until mixture resembles fine bread crumbs. Stir in the sugar and dates. Using a round-bladed knife, stir in the milk and mix until mixture forms a ball. Toss mixture onto a lightly floured board and knead until smooth. Roll mixture to 15mm thickness and using a scone cutter, cut into rounds. Place scones close together on prepared baking slide and brush with milk.
3. Bake for 15 minutes or until the scones sound hollow when tapped. Serve spread with Flora pro-activ.

Makes 12-15.

Blueberry Muffins

Preparation Time: 15 minutes
Cooking Time: 15-20 minutes

Flora pro-activ, melted, for brushing tin

1 $^3/_4$ cups self-raising flour

1 teaspoon baking powder

$^1/_2$ teaspoon ground cinnamon

$^1/_4$ cup caster sugar

$^1/_2$ cup blueberries

60g ($^1/_4$ cup) Flora pro-activ, extra, melted

1 cup reduced-fat milk

1 egg, lightly beaten

1 teaspoon vanilla essence

1. Pre-heat oven to 200°C. Brush a 1 x 12-cup non-stick muffin tin with melted Flora pro-activ.
2. Sift flour, baking powder and cinnamon into a bowl, mix in sugar and blueberries. In another bowl combine extra Flora pro-activ, milk, egg and vanilla. Using a wooden spoon, mix the Flora pro-activ mixture into the dry ingredients until just combined (16 strokes). Spoon mixture into prepared tin.
3. Bake for 15-20 minutes or until a warmed skewer inserted in the centre comes out clean. Serve warm or cold spread with Flora pro-activ.

Makes 12.

Lemon Poppy Seed Muffins

Preparation Time: 15 minutes
Cooking Time: 15-20 minutes

Flora pro-activ, melted, for brushing tin

1 ³/₄ cups self-raising flour

1 teaspoon baking powder

¹/₄ cup caster sugar

1 tablespoon poppy seeds

1 tablespoon grated lemon rind

60g (¹/₄ cup) Flora pro-activ, extra, melted

250mL (1 cup) reduced-fat milk

1 egg, lightly beaten

20mL (1 tablespoon) lemon juice

1. Pre-heat oven to 200°C. Brush a 1 x 12-cup non-stick muffin tin with melted Flora pro-activ.
2. Sift flour and baking powder into a bowl, mix in sugar, poppy seeds and lemon rind. In another bowl, combine extra melted Flora pro-activ, milk, egg and lemon juice. Using a wooden spoon, mix the Flora pro-activ mixture into the dry ingredients until just combined (16 strokes). Spoon mixture into prepared tin.
3. Bake for 15-20 minutes or until a warmed skewer inserted in the centre comes out clean. Serve warm or cold spread with Flora pro-activ.

Makes 12.

Carrot and Walnut Loaf

Preparation Time: 15 minutes
Cooking Time: 45 minutes

1 ³/₄ cups self-raising flour

1 teaspoon baking powder

1 teaspoon ground cinnamon

¹/₂ cup firmly packed brown sugar

1 cup grated carrot

¹/₂ cup finely chopped walnuts

125g (¹/₂ cup) Flora pro-activ, melted

2 eggs, lightly beaten

125mL (¹/₂ cup) reduced-fat milk

¹/₂ teaspoon vanilla essence

1. Pre-heat oven to 180°C. Line a 23 x 13cm loaf tin with baking paper.
2. Sift flour, baking powder and cinnamon into a mixing bowl. Add brown sugar, carrot, walnuts, melted Flora pro-activ, eggs, milk and vanilla. Mix, with a wooden spoon, until well combined. Place mixture into prepared tin.
3. Bake for 45 minutes or until a warmed skewer inserted in the centre comes out clean. Allow to cool in tin for 5 minutes before transferring to a wire cooling tray. Cool. Serve, sliced, spread with Flora pro-activ.

Makes 1 loaf.

Olive and Sun-dried Tomato Bread

Preparation Time: 15 minutes
Cooking Time: 45 minutes

2 cups self-raising flour

¹/₄ cup sliced black olives

2 tablespoons finely chopped sun-dried tomatoes

60g (¹/₄ cup) Flora pro-activ, melted

2 eggs, lightly beaten

165mL (²/₃ cup) reduced-fat milk

1. Pre-heat oven to 190°C. Line a 23 x 13cm loaf tin with baking paper.
2. Sift flour into a mixing bowl, add olives, sun-dried tomatoes, melted Flora pro-activ, eggs and milk. Mix with a wooden spoon, until well combined. Place mixture into prepared tin.
3. Bake for 45 minutes or until a warmed skewer inserted in the centre comes out clean. Allow to cool in tin for 5 minutes before transferring to a wire cooling tray. Cool. Serve, sliced, spread with Flora pro-activ.

Makes 1 loaf.

Apricot Pudding

Preparation Time: 15 minutes
Cooking Time: 25 minutes

1-2 teaspoons Flora pro-activ, melted

1 cup self-raising flour

$^1/_2$ teaspoon baking powder

$^1/_4$ cup caster sugar

60g ($^1/_4$ cup) Flora pro-activ, extra, melted

2 eggs, lightly beaten

125mL ($^1/_2$ cup) reduced-fat milk

$^1/_2$ teaspoon vanilla essence

1 x 425g can apricot halves, drained

Icing sugar for garnish

Berries for serving

1. Pre-heat oven to 200°C. Brush a round, 1-litre capacity baking dish with melted Flora pro-activ.
2. Sift flour and baking powder into a mixing bowl. Add sugar, extra melted Flora pro-activ, eggs, milk and vanilla. Mix with a wooden spoon, until well combined. Place mixture into prepared dish.
3. Bake for 5 minutes, open oven and drop apricot halves, hollow-side down, into cake mixture. Bake for a further 20 minutes or until a warmed skewer inserted in the centre comes out clean and the pudding is golden. Cool slightly and serve, sprinkled with icing sugar accompanied by fresh berries.

Serves 6-8.

Moist Date Cake

Preparation Time: 15 minutes
Cooking Time: 30 minutes

³/₄ cup pitted dates, chopped

185mL (³/₄ cup) water

1 teaspoon bicarbonate of soda

60g (¹/₄ cup) Flora pro-activ

¹/₂ cup caster sugar

1 egg, lightly beaten

¹/₂ teaspoon vanilla essence

1 cup self-raising flour

Low-fat yoghurt for serving

1. Pre-heat oven to 190°C. Line a 20cm round cake tin with baking paper.
2. Place dates and water in a saucepan and bring to the boil. Remove from the heat and stir in the bicarbonate of soda, set aside. Cream Flora pro-activ and sugar with an electric hand-held mixer until light. Add egg and vanilla and mix well. Fold in the flour and dates. Place mixture into prepared tin.
3. Bake for 30 minutes or until a warm skewer inserted in the centre comes out clean. Cool in tin for 5 minutes before transferring to a wire cooling rack. Serve sliced accompanied with yoghurt.

Serves 6-8.

Oat and Sultana Biscuits

Preparation Time: 15 minutes
Cooking Time: 20 minutes

85g (¹/₃ cup) Flora pro-activ

¹/₃ cup white sugar

1 egg, lightly beaten

2-3 drops vanilla essence

²/₃ cup sultanas

1 cup self-raising flour

²/₃ cup rolled oats

1. Pre-heat oven to 180°C. Line baking trays with baking paper.
2. Cream Flora pro-activ and sugar, with a hand-held electric mixer, until light and fluffy. Add egg and vanilla and mix well. Fold in sultanas and flour. Drop teaspoonfuls of mixture into oats and roll into balls. Place onto prepared trays, pressing down lightly with fingertips, allowing room for spreading.
3. Bake for 20 minutes or until golden. Allow to go cold on baking trays. Store in an airtight container.

Makes approximately 24.

Dessert Ideas

Serve fruits in season fresh, poached or baked.
Serve low-fat plain or flavoured yoghurt with desserts.

Apple and Pear Crumble

Preparation Time: 15 minutes
Cooking Time: 15 minutes

2 Granny Smith apples, peeled, cored and chopped

1 Packham pear, peeled and chopped

$^1/_3$ cup raisins

$^1/_2$ stick cinnamon

185mL ($^3/_4$ cup) water

$^1/_2$ cup self-raising flour

$^1/_4$ teaspoon cinnamon

2 tablespoons brown sugar

40g (2 tablespoons) Flora pro-activ

1. Pre-heat oven to 210°C .
2. Place apple, pear, raisins, cinnamon stick and water in a saucepan, cover and cook until tender. Drain. Place fruit into a 1-litre capacity ovenproof dish. Sift flour and cinnamon into a bowl and stir in the sugar. Using your fingertips, rub Flora pro-activ into the mixture and sprinkle over the fruit.
3. Bake for 15 minutes or until golden. Serve with low-fat yoghurt.

Serves 4-6.

> **Hint:** Use plums, cherries or apricots when in season for crumbles. Recipe may be cooked and served in individual size dishes.

Quick & Easy

5 THINGS TO DO WITH A CAN OF PINK SALMON

Add to Roasted Vegetable Lasagne (see recipe page 141).

Add to heated pasta sauce and serve over cooked pasta.

Add to Basic White Sauce (see recipe page 151), add chopped chives or shallots and serve over rice.

Add to Mixed Lettuce and Baby Spinach Salad with Herb Dressing (see page 125).

Add to a Chinese Cabbage, Carrot and Chives with Asian Dressing (see page 125).

5 THINGS TO DO WITH A BOTTLE OF PASTA SAUCE

Add to Chunky Vegetable Soup (see recipe page 128).

Add to Mediterranean Soup (see recipe page 137).

Add to Roasted Vegetable Lasagne (see recipe page 141).

Heat sauce and serve with Roast Lamb with Rosemary with Creamed Roasted Garlic (see recipe page 130).

Heat with a can of drained butter beans or kidney beans and serve over pasta, sprinkled with parsley.

Relax and Enjoy

5 THINGS TO DO WITH A CUP OF TEA

Add honey and lemon juice to taste.

Add a cinnamon stick and brown sugar to taste.

Add 2-3 drops of vanilla essence and sugar to taste.

Add grated green ginger, lemon juice and honey to taste.

Add mint leaves, cinnamon and sugar to taste.

Flora pro-activ is the registered Trademark of Unilever Australia Limited

74 Edinburgh Road, Marrickville. NSW 2204

Glossary

Angina Chest pain brought on by exercise. Caused by insufficient blood supply to the heart due to narrowed coronary arteries.

Antioxidants Substances which inactivate free radicals, thereby limiting oxidation in the body. The body makes some antioxidants and obtains others through food.

Arrhythmia A breakdown in the normal, steady beating of the heart. In mild cases may cause 'heart flutter'; in severe cases can cause the heart to stop beating.

Atherosclerosis The slow build up of cholesterol and other substances (plaque) on the walls of the coronary arteries. Causes narrowing of the arteries which can restrict blood flow.

Cholesterol A waxy substance present in foods of animal origin. Cholesterol can also be made in the body and performs many useful roles. Although always present in the blood, cholesterol increases the risk of heart disease when it occurs at high levels.

'Coronary' See heart attack

Coronary arteries Blood vessels which supply the heart with oxygen.

Coronary heart disease Restricted blood flow through the coronary arteries. The result of atherosclerosis. Causes angina and may lead to a heart attack.

DHA See omega-3

EPA See omega-3

Essential fatty acids Two polyunsaturated fatty acids which are essential nutrients in the diet. They also have a blood cholesterol-lowering effect. Seed oils are especially rich sources.

Flavonoids Powerful antioxidants found in red wine and tea.

Folate B vitamin which lowers the level of homocysteine in the blood.

Free radicals Unbalanced, potentially dangerous molecules formed in the body. Antioxidants quench free radicals and limit their damage.

HDL-cholesterol Cholesterol which has been picked up from the body's cells and is passing through the blood back to the liver. Often referred to as 'good' cholesterol as it is protective against heart disease.

Heart attack Life-threatening event caused by the complete blockage of a coronary artery, which prevents oxygen reaching part of the heart. The immediate cause is usually a blot clot, which forms when a plaque in the coronary artery tears apart.

Homocysteine A substance produced in the body as a normal part of metabolism, which increases the risk of heart disease when it occurs at high levels in the blood.

LDL-cholesterol The 'bad' cholesterol in the blood, so-called because it is destined to be deposited in the walls of blood vessels. High levels of LDL-cholesterol in the blood are linked with increased risk of heart disease.

Monounsaturated fatty acids A major component of fat in the diet, found in a variety of foods, notably olive and canola oils. Has a neutral effect on blood cholesterol.

Omega-3 A type of polyunsaturated fatty acid. Comes in plant and marine forms, both of which are thought to be protective against heart disease. The marine form has components EPA and DHA, which are responsible for the protective effects of fish against heart disease.

Oxidation A damaging process in the body caused by free radicals. Oxidation is kept in check by antioxidants.

Plant sterols Natural, cholesterol-like substances found in all whole, plant foods. Plant sterols have a strong blood cholesterol-lowering effect when consumed in sufficient amounts.

Plaque A collection of cholesterol and other substances on the wall of a coronary artery; the end result of atherosclerosis. The rupture of a plaque leads to a heart attack.

Polyunsaturated fatty acids A major component of fat in the diet, found in a variety of foods. Includes the essential fatty acids, which have a blood cholesterol-lowering effect and marine omega-3 which is protective against heart disease in other ways.

Risk factors Factors which increase the risk of heart disease. The three major risk factors are high blood cholesterol, high blood pressure and smoking. Other important risk factors include family history of heart disease, overweight and diabetes.

Saturated fatty acids A major component of fat in the diet, found in a variety of foods, especially dairy foods, meat and baked goods. The major cholesterol-raising agent the diet.

Trans fatty acids A minor component of fat in the diet, found in dairy foods, meat and some baked goods. Recently removed from most margarines.

References

(1)   Kannel WB, Castelli WP, Gordon T et al. Serum cholesterol, lipoproteins and risk of coronary heart disease: the Framingham Study. Ann Intern Med 1971;74:1-12.

(2)   Stamler J, Wentworth D, Neaton JD. Is relationship between serum cholesterol and risk of premature death from coronary heart disease continuous and graded? Findings in 356,222 primary screenees of the Multiple Risk Factor Intervention Trial (MRFIT). JAMA 1986;256:2823-2828.

(3)   Scandinavian Simvastatin Survival Study Group. Randomised trial of cholesterol lowering in 4444 patients with coronary heart disease: the Scandinavian Simvastatin Survival Study. Lancet 1994;344:1383-1389.

(4)   Shepherd J, Cobbe SM, Ford I et al. Prevention of coronary heart disease with pravastatin in men with hypercholesterolaemia. N Engl J Med 1995;333:1301-1307.

(5)   Sacks FM, Pfeffer MA, Moye LA et al. The effect of pravastatin on coronary events after myocardial infarction in patients with average cholesterol levels. N Engl J Med 1996;335:1001-1009.

(6)   The LIPID Study Group. Prevention of cardiovascular events and death with pravastatin in patients with coronary heart disease and a broad range of initial cholesterol levels. N Engl J Med 1998;339:1349-57.

(7)   Weststrate JA, Meijer GW. Plant sterol enriched margarines and reduction of plasma total- and LDL-cholesterol concentrations in normocholesterolaemic and mildly hypercholesterolaemic subjects. Eur J Clin Nutr 1998;52:334-343.

(8)   Hendriks HFJ, Weststrate JA, van Vliet T et al. Spreads enriched with three different levels of vegetable oil sterols and the degree of cholesterol lowering in normocholesterolaemic and mildly hypercholesterolaemic subjects. Eur J Clin Nutr 1999;53:319-327.

(9)   Clifton P, Noakes M, Record I et al. An increase in dietary carotenoids is effective in preventing the reduction in plasma carotenoid concentrations from plant sterol enriched margarines. (submitted for publication).

(10)   Baker VA, Hepburn PA, Kennedy SJ et al. Safety evaluation of phytosterol esters. Part 1. Assessment of oestrogenicity using a combination of in vivo and in vitro assays. Food Chem Toxicol 1999;37:13-22.

(11)   Hepburn PA, Horners SA, Smith M. Safety evaluation of phytosterol esters. Part 2. Subchronic 90-day oral toxicity study on phytosterol-esters – a novel functional food. Food Chem Toxicol 1999;37:521-532.

(12)   Waalkens-Berendsen DH, Wolterbeek APM, Wijnands MVW, et al. Safety evaluation of phytosterol esters. Part 3. Two-generation reproduction studyin rats with phytosterol esters - a novel functional food. Food Chem Toxicol 1999;37:683-696.

(13)   Weststrate JA, Ayesh R, Bauer-Plank C et al. Safety evaluation of phytosterol esters. Part 4. Faecal concentrations of bile acids and neutral sterols in healthy normolipaemic volunteers consuming a controlled diet either with or without a phytosterol ester-enriched margarine. Food Chem Toxicol 1999;37:1063-1071.

(14)   Ayesh R, Weststrate JA, Drewitt PN et al. Safety evaluation of phytosterol esters. Part 5. Faecal short-chain fatty acid and microflora content, faecal bacterial enzyme activity and plasma female sex hormones in healthy normolipaemic volunteers consuming a controlled diet either with or without a phytosterol ester-enriched margarine. Food Chem Toxicol 1999;37:1127-1138.

(15)   Cordain L, Brand-Miller J, Boyd Eaton S et al. Plant to animal subsistence ratios and macronutrient energy estimations in world wide hunter-gatherer diets. Am J Clin Nutr 2000;71 (in press).

(16)   Keys A, Anderson JT, Grande F. Prediction of blood cholesterol responses of man to changes in fats in the diet. Lancet 1957;2:959-966.

(17)   Hegsted DM, McGandy RB, Myers SM et al. Quantitative effects of dietary fat on blood cholesterol in man. Am J Clin Nutr 1965;14:776-787.

(18)   Renaud S, de Lorgeril M. Wine, alcohol, platelets and the French paradox for coronary heart disease. Lancet 1992;339:1523-1526.

(19)   Mensink RP, Katan MB. Effects of dietary trans fatty acids on high-density and low-density lipoprotein cholesterol levels in healthy subjects. N Engl J Med 1990;323:439-445.

(20)   Hu FB, Stampfer MJ, Manson JE et al. Dietary saturated fats and their food sources in relation to the risk of coronary heart disease in women. Am J Clin Nutr 1999;70:1001-1008.

(21)   National Heart Foundation of Australia. A review of the relationship between dietary fat and cardiovascular disease. Aust J Nutr Diet 1999;56(4 Suppl):S5-S22.

(22)   Keys A, Menotti A, Karvonen MJ et al. The diet and the 15-year death rate in the Seven Countries Study. Am J Epidemiol 1986;124:903-915.

(23)   Keys A. Olive oil and heart disease [letter]. Lancet 1987;1(April 25):983-984.

(24)   Rudel LL, Parks JS, Sawyer, JK. Compared with dietary monounsaturated and saturated fat, polyunsaturated fat protects African green monkeys from coronary artery atherosclerosis. Arterioscler Thromb Vasc Biol 1995;15:2101-2110.

(25)   Fraser GE, Sabate J, Beeson WL et al. A possible protective effect of nut consumption on risk of coronary heart disease: the Adventist Health Study. Arch Intern Med 1992; 152:1416-1424.

(26)   Kushi LH, Folsom AR, Prineas RJ et al. Dietary antioxidant vitamins and death from coronary heart disease in postmenopausal women. N Engl J Med 1996;334:1156-1162.

(27)   Hu FB, Stampfer MJ, Manson JE et al. Frequent nut consumption and risk of coronary heart disease in women: prospective cohort study. BMJ 1998;317:1341-1345.

(28)   Allred JB. Too much of a good thing? JADA 1995;95:417-418.

References

(29)   Steinberg D, Parthasarathy S, Carew TE et al. Beyond cholesterol: modifications of low-density lipoprotein that increase its atherogenicity. N Engl J Med 1989;320:915-924.

(30)   Gey KF, Moser UK, Jordan P et al. Increased risk of cardiovascular disease at suboptimal plasma concentrations of essential antioxidants: an epidemiological update with special attention to carotene and vitamin C. Am J Clin Nutr 1993;57(suppl):787S-797S.

(31)   Bellizzi MC, Franklin MF, Duthie GG et al. Vitamin E and coronary heart disease: the European paradox. Eur J Clin Nutr 1994;48:822-831.

(32)   Stampfer MJ, Hennekens CH, Manson JE et al. Vitamin E consumption and the risk of coronary disease in women. N Engl J Med 1993;328:1444-1449.

(33)   Rimm EB, Stampfer MJ, Ascherio A et al. Vitamin E consumption and the risk of coronary heart disease in men. N Engl J Med 1993;328:1450-1456.

(34)   Hertog MGL, Kromhout D, Aravanis C et al. Flanonoid intake and long-term risk of coronary heart disease and cancer in the Seven Countries Study. Arch Intern Med 1995;155:381-386.

(35)   Hertog MGL, Feskens EJM, Hollman PCH et al. Dietary antioxidant flavonoids and risk of coronary heart disease: the Zutphen Elderly Study. Lancet 1993;342:1007-1011.

(36)   Heinonen OP, Huttunen JK, Albanes D et al. The effect of vitamin E and beta carotene on the incidence of lung cancer and other cancers in male smokers. N Engl J Med 1994;330:1029-1035.

(37)   Omenn GS, Goodman GE, Thornquist MD et al. Effects of combination beta carotene and vitamin A on lung cancer and cardiovascular disease. N Engl J Med 1996;334:1150-1155.

(38)   Holman CDJ, English DR, Milne E et al. Meta-analysis of alcohol and all-cause mortality: a validation of NHMRC recommendations. MJA 1996;164:141-145.

(39)   Kromhout D, Bosschieter EB, de Lezenne Coulander C. The inverse relation between fish consumption and 20-year mortality from coronary heart disease. N Engl J Med 1985;312:1205-1209.

(40)   Daviglas ML, Stamler J, Orencia AJ et al. Fish consumption and the 30-year risk of fatal myocardial infarction. N Engl J Med 1997;336:1046-1053.

(41)   Burr ML, Fehily AM, Gilbert JF et al. Effects of changes in fat, fish and fibre intakes on death and myocardial reinfarction: Diet and Reinfarction Trial (DART). Lancet 1989;2:757-761.

(42)   McLennan PL, Abeywardena MY, Charnock JS. Dietary fish oil prevents ventricular fibrillation following coronary artery occlusion and reperfusion. Am Heart J 1988;116:709-717.

(43)   de Lorgeril M, Renaud S, Mamelle N et al. Mediterranean alpha-linolenic acid-rich diet in secondary prevention of coronary heart disease. Lancet 1994;343:1454-1459.

(44)   Boushey CJ, Beresford SA, Omenn GS et al. A quantitative assessment of plasma homocysteine as a risk factor for vascular disease. JAMA 1995;274:1049-1057.

(45)   Consumer Science Program, CSIRO Human Nutrition. Beverage Consumption: Results from the 1995/6 National Nutrition Survey. A report for Unilever Australia.

(46)   Grubben MJ, Boers GH, Blom HJ et al. Unfiltered coffee increases plasma homocysteine concentrations in healthy volunteers: a randomised trial. Am J Clin Nutr 2000;71:480-484.

(47)   Rimm EB, Ascherio A, Giovannucci E et al. Vegetable, fruit and cereal fibre intake and risk of coronary heart disease among men. JAMA 1996;275:447-451.

(48)   Liu S, Stampfer MJ, Hu FB et al. Whole-grain consumption and risk of coronary heart disease: results from the Nurses Health Study. Am J Clin Nutr 1999;70:412-419.

(49)   Svetkey LP, Simons-Morton D, Vollmer WM et al. Effects of dietary patterns on blood pressure: subgroup analysis of the Dietary Approaches to Stop Hypertension (DASH) randomised clinical trial. Arch Intern Med 1999;159:285-293.

(50)   Dattilo AM, Kris-Etherton PM. Effects of weight reduction on blood lipids and lipoproteins: a meta-analysis. Am J Clin Nutr 1992;56:320-328.

(51)   Prentice AM, Jebb SA. Obesity in Britain: gluttony or sloth? BMJ 1995;311:437-439.

Index

A
alcohol 62-66
and blood pressure 78
beneficial effects 62-64
damaging effects 64-65
and HDL-cholesterol 63-64
alpha-carotene 55
angina 13
animal foods 93-94
antioxidants 52-61, 64
enzymes 54
fat-soluble 54-55
in red wine 64
in tea 59-60
supplements 60-61
water-soluble 56-57
arrhythmia 70-71
atherosclerosis 13

B
beta-carotene 55-56, 57
blood pressure 15, 77-78
butter 36-39, 42

C
calcium 79,94
carotenoids 55-56, 57
cholesterol 11-21
absorption from gut 17, 24-25
bad cholesterol 18-19
dietary (in food) 49-51
factors affecting 19-20
good cholesterol 18-19
HDL-cholesterol 17-19
LDL-cholesterol 17-19
oxidation 53-54, 57-58
transport system 16-19
clot 13
coronary arteries 12-13
coronary heart disease 13-15

D
DHA 68
diabetes 31-32
dietary quality 87-89

E
eggs 50-51
empty calories 87-88
EPA 68
essential fatty acids 34-35
exercise 81-85

F
fat 34-48
animal fats 35-39

cholesterol-lowering 39-41
cholesterol-raising 37-39
fatty acids 34-37
fat-soluble vitamins 35
fat-soluble antioxidants 54-56
low-fat diets 44-45, 47
monounsaturated 42-43
overweight 47, 80-91
polyunsaturated 39-41
saturated 35-38
trans fatty acids 39
fibre 75-77
fish 67-73
flavonoids 56-57
folate 74-75
free radicals 53-54

G
glycaemic index 45
HDL-cholesterol 17-19
effects of alcohol 63
effects of fats 44-45

H
heart 12
heart disease 13-15
heart attack 13
homocysteine 74-75

I
iron 93-94
isoflavones 77

J
J curve 65-66

L
LDL-cholesterol 17-19
effects of fats 37-43
effects of plant sterols 26-29
low-fat diets 44-45, 47
lycopene 55-57

M
marine omega-3 68-73
amounts in fish 69
arrhythmia 70-71
meat 93-94
monounsaturated fats 42-43
effects on cholesterol 42-43

N
nuts 45-46

O
olive oil 42-43
omega balance 72
omega-3 68-72
marine omega-3 68-72
plant omega-3   71-72

overweight 80-91
causes 81-84
effects on cholesterol 80-81
effects on blood pressure 80
exercise 81, 84-85
weight gain/weight loss 82-83
oxidation 53-54, 57-58

P
physical activity 81, 84-85
plant sterols 8-9, 22-33
discovery 25-26
effects on LDL 26-29
effects on HDL 27
mode of action 24-25
research studies 27-29
side effects 30-31
sources 23-24
plaque 13
polyphenols 56-57
in tea 59-60
in wine 64
polyunsaturated fats 36-41
effects on cholesterol 39-41
marine omega-3 68-72
plant omega-3   71-72
potassium 79
prawns 50, 107
p/s ratio 40-41

R
risk factors 14-15

S
salt 77-79
saturated fats 35-38
effects on cholesterol 37-38
shopping 115
smoking 15, 56
sodium 77-79
soy 77
soy protein 77
starch 44-45
sterols 8-9, 22-33
animal sterols 16, 23
plant sterols 8-9, 22-33
sugar 87-88
sunflower oil 37, 42, 54-55, 58

T
tea 59-60
trans fatty acids 39

V
variety 92-95
vitamin C 56
vitamin E 54-55, 57-59

W
whole foods 76
wholegrains 75-76

Recipe Index

A
Apple and Pear Crumble 161
Apricot Pudding 158
Asian Beef Noodle Soup 138

B
Baking:
Apple and Pear Crumble 161
Apricot Pudding 158
Blueberry Muffins 154
Carrot and Walnut Loaf 156
Date Scones 153
Herb Scones 152
Lemon Poppy Seed Muffins 155
Moist Date Cake 159
Oat and Sultana Biscuits 160
Olive and Sun-dried Tomato Bread 157
Basic Stir-fry Vegetables 148
Beef:
Asian Beef Noodle Soup 138
Beef Casserole 132
Beef Stew with Herb Dumplings 136
Stir-fry Asian Beef Noodles 143
Blueberry Muffins 154

C
Carrot and Walnut Loaf 156
Chicken:
Chicken and Corn Soup 127
Chicken and Vegetable Curry 131
Honey Teriyaki Chicken and Vegetable Stir-fry 142
Pumpkin Risotto with Chicken 139
Chunky Vegetable Soup 128
Creamy Mushrooms with Fettuccine 146

D
Date Scones 153

F
Fish:
Pan-fried Fish Fillets 135
Smoked Cod with Onion and Parsley Sauce 134
Sun-dried Tomato and Salmon Cutlet Parcels 144
Flavoured spreads: 123
Apricot and Almond
Garlic

Herb
Herb and Garlic
Olive
Onion and Rosemary
Pizza
Roasted Capsicum
Roasted Walnut
Sun-dried Tomato

H
Herb Scones 152
Honey Teriyaki Chicken and Vegetable Stir-fry 142
Hot and Tasty Breads 122

L
Lamb:
Marinated Lamb Cutlets 145
Moroccan Lamb with Prunes, Almonds and Couscous 140
Roast Lamb with Rosemary and Creamed Roasted Garlic 130
Lemon Poppy Seed Muffins 155

M
Marinated Lamb Cutlets 145
Mashed Potatoes 149
Mediterranean Soup 137
Moist Date Cake 159
Moroccan Lamb with Prunes, Almonds and Couscous 140

O
Oat and Sultana Biscuits 160
Olive and Sun-dried Tomato Bread 157

P
Pan-fried Fish Fillets 135
Pumpkin Risotto with Chicken 139

R
Roast Lamb with Rosemary and Creamed Roasted Garlic 130
Roasted Vegetable Lasagne 141
Roast Vegetables 147

S
Salads: 125
Asparagus, Red Capsicum and Toasted Almond
Chinese Cabbage, Carrot and Chives
Cooked Chicken, Cos Lettuce, Yellow Capsicum and Croutons
Cooked New Potatoes, Shallots and Mint
Mesclun, Roma Tomatoes, Spanish Onion
Mixed Lettuce and Baby Spinach
Mushroom, Shallot and Walnut

Prawn, Pineapple and Mignonette Lettuce
Rare Roast Beef, Coriander, Cherry Tomato and Lettuce
Tomato and Basil

Salad Dressings: 124
Asian
Basic dressing
Herb
Italian
Sandwich Fillings and Toppings: 126
Avocado and Sweet Chilli
Carrot, Sultana and Walnuts
Ham, Lettuce and Mustard
Lamb, Mint Sauce and Baby Spinach
Roast Beef, Tomato and Pickle
Salmon, Capers and Dill
Sardine and Onion
Shaved Chicken with Mango Chutney
Shaved Turkey, Alfalfa Sprouts and Cranberry Sauce
Tuna, Lettuce and Tomato
Sauces: 151
Asparagus and Capsicum
Basic White Sauce
Chicken and Creamed Corn
Dijon Mustard, Honey and Walnut
Ham and Mushroom
Herbed Lemon
Olive and Caper
Roasted Vegetables and Pine Nuts

Salmon and Shallot
Sun-dried Tomato
Tuna and Parsley

Soups:
Asian Beef Noodle Soup 138
Chicken and Corn Soup 127
Chunky Vegetable Soup 128
Mediterranean Soup 137
Smoked Cod with Onion and Parsley Sauce 134
Steamed Vegetables 150
Stir-fry Asian Beef Noodles 143
Sun-dried Tomato and Salmon Cutlet Parcels 144

T
Traditional and Open Sandwiches 126
Tuna and Carrot Pasta Bake 133
U

V
Veal:
Veal in Tomato and Onion Gravy 129
Vegetable dishes:
Basic Stir-fry Vegetables 148
Creamy Mushrooms with Fettuccine 146
Mashed Potatoes   149
Roasted Vegetable Lasagne 141
Roast Vegetables 147
Steamed Vegetables 150